SMALL DOSES OF AWARENESS

SMALL DOSES OF AWARENESS

A MICRODOSING COMPANION

GUIDED JOURNAL

BY SHIN YU PAI & AMY WONG HOPE, MSW, LCSW

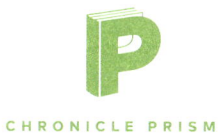

CHRONICLE PRISM

HOW TO USE THIS JOURNAL 6
NOTES FROM THE AUTHORS 8
INTRODUCTION 18

Week One - 35
Creating Safety

Week Two - 47
Leaning into the Senses

Week Three - 59
How I See Me

Week Four - 71
How I Connect with the World

Week Five - 83
What I've Assumed to Be True

Week Six - 95
Where I Belong

Week Seven - 107
The Art of Not Doing

Week Eight - 119
The Art of Doing

Week Nine - 131
*My Foundation and
Who Shaped It*

Week Ten - 143
What I Want to Anchor In

Week Eleven - 155
*Holding the Self in the
World Differently*

Week Twelve and Beyond - 167
After Microdosing

AFTERWORD 180
BIBLIOGRAPHY 184
RESOURCES 186
ABOUT THE AUTHORS 188
ACKNOWLEDGMENTS 190

HOW TO USE THIS JOURNAL

Journaling about your experiences with microdosing can help you reflect on thoughts and insights that arise for you throughout your journey. Recording your observations and feelings is one way to get to know your own mind and to reimagine the narratives that you've absorbed about yourself.

While microdosing can set the stage for resetting behaviors and beliefs, journaling can be the self-care and wellness practice that helps you make sense of your experiences. By writing, you can become more aware of negative patterns and self-talk that can get in the way of deeper experience and connection. And by identifying these patterns, you can move toward choosing other ways of being in the world, more fully integrating what you've learned.

This journal offers short exploratory essays and guided questions alternating with Insights and Observations log pages where you can process how you are adjusting to your microdosing experiences. You'll have the opportunity to bring awareness to your mind and body over time, enabling you to notice where shifts may be happening for you.

In this book, we sometimes share realizations that are specific to our cultural experiences as Asian American women. We share openly and vulnerably about cultural trauma to invite you to explore your own subtle awareness of where inequity has impacted your life.

All journeys have a beginning, middle, and end. We've organized each week by key themes that gradually move into a deeper space over time. As you travel through your experience and this journal, you'll explore opening into curiosity, coming into deeper awareness, and integrating what you've learned into your everyday life and your experiences.

While this journal is written to serve as a personal guide for individual exploration, it can also be beneficial to share this practice with a friend or partner who is on their own journey and with whom you wish to discuss the experience of microdosing.

Lastly, some journals are structured as workbooks, a program to work through once. Use this book in whatever way works for you. You may find value in revisiting certain inquiry questions or completed journal entries. Whether you are coming back to prompts that may offer new answers with time or turning back to lessons learned along your path—this journal exists to hold the space for your experiences.

NOTES FROM THE AUTHORS

UNDOING THE LONELINESS

Eighteen months into the pandemic, I woke up one morning and measured out a microdose of pulverized mushroom into a small ceramic cup, poured hot water onto the powder, and brewed a medicinal tea. I'd planned this moment for a day when my eight-year-old son would be at school. I'd taken the day off from my nonprofit job and blocked out the time on my calendar to be free of distractions. I silenced my cell phone ringer, turned off text messaging, and told my partner that I'd see him in a few hours.

It had been a brutal summer of rolling heat waves and climate fires that made it necessary to stay indoors. My emotions and nervous system had been frazzled by the ongoing news reports of hate crimes against Asian American women and elders and the seemingly endless wait for a coronavirus vaccine for children. Deprived of the ability to go for a daily run alone or to de-stress from work by going out into nature, my mental health began to suffer. The CBD oil that I'd occasionally use after being off antidepressants for a year had lost its effectiveness in managing my long-term depression, and I was ready to try something new.

Though I'd taken LSD and psilocybin a handful of times throughout my high school and college years, I wasn't sure what to expect this time. I addressed my anxiety by reading everything I could get my hands on about microdosing and by speaking with friends who'd experimented with mushrooms, MDMA, and LSD. By arming myself with information, I hoped to find some sense of control or confidence as I embarked on my journey, but there were still unknowns.

Forty-five minutes after drinking the mushroom tea, I looked out the picture window of my backyard office and noticed the color of the pine trees deepening in intensity as they swayed in the breeze against the bright blue sky. My mind slowed down, and the emotional "stuckness" that I had felt inside of me all year dissipated. I felt more like myself. This was significant because a sense of well-being had felt out of reach for so long. It took me a long moment to feel it sink in.

Psilocybin isn't yet legal in most places, and it felt taboo to talk openly with most people about my new experiences with microdosing. The person who introduced me to microdosing didn't want to coach me through the experience. They were starting a full-time corporate job and needed to limit their commitments. I had a preexisting friendship with this person, and we didn't want to complicate that relationship. They were deliberate in their parting words, when they warned me that without coaching, the benefits of microdosing would fail to take root. Without someone to integrate the experience with me—someone who had undergone the psychedelic journey with mushrooms firsthand—I'd be lost at sea.

    The sense of abandonment and despair that I felt nearly led me to give up my experiment. But I'd been thoughtful about setting up a community of care to support me. A month before microdosing, I reconnected with my psychotherapist and asked if we could set up a few sessions that would support integration of my experiences and help me navigate the psychedelic space. I'd taken a long break from talk therapy by then, but combining microdosing with neuroplasticity work made sense to me. My therapist had supported others on their microdosing journeys and agreed to resume seeing me, and our sessions together focused on bringing more mindfulness and curiosity to each microdosing experience.

    It was in those early days of exploring microdosing that the idea of a guided journal first came to me. I began recording my intentions and experiences in a notebook on both dosing and nondosing days when I wanted to record the effects of microdosing in my system. I wrote down my realizations and physical and emotional changes every day and logged the particulars of my microdosing days. But I wanted a more structured space where I could be more thoughtful about my experiences with psychedelics, a place where I could extract my own learnings and make new discoveries by directing my mind toward contemplation.

    When I started thinking about creating this journal, I reached out to my friend Amy Wong Hope. Amy and I met nearly twenty years ago in Boston, when she signed up to take a poetry class I taught. We stayed in touch, and I kept an eye on her many moves. She left a career in the corporate sector to pursue a path of healing arts that took her to New Mexico—a place where I also felt a strong sense of creative and spiritual community. In Santa Fe, we reconnected and picked up our friendship where we left off. We'd both been on our own separate healing journeys, and yet so many of the places that we'd arrived in understanding our own experiences in the world resonated with one another, including the tools and the medicine that we used to take us to those places.

This book is the microdosing journal that I wanted most in those early days of self-discovery to combat the loneliness. I wrote it with a friend who also understands that interior terrain and knows the power of asking questions of your mind so that your soul can echo back. It's in this spirit that we offer this book to you. It was born of our own experience and deep belief in every individual's capacity to be their own trusted guide and healer.

—*Shin Yu Pai*

ARRIVING AT THE SUBTLE

My first experiences with psychedelics were macrodoses, not microdoses. These experiences brought me a powerful new set of lenses through which I was able to see how shame had driven my lifelong feeling of anxiety. Though psychotherapy helped me tremendously through the years, the insights received through psychedelics were profound. They were both a microscope and a telescope simultaneously—a close-up and a wide-angle view at the same time. It felt like a superpower. I saw how my overcompensating behaviors, such as being a people pleaser and perfectionist, were born out of fear and shame. I saw how they had prevented me from living with presence, full authenticity, and pleasure.

The problem is that groundbreaking insights alone don't ensure integration of new learning. *Integration* is the process of unifying these insights with action—embodying the changes in behavior, emotions, and thought patterns we need to feel whole. And while this may seem like a simple thing, changing our behavior or identity is complex. Nowhere is this truer than in the process of integration.

The undoing of shame required a painstaking, yearslong commitment. Before I started microdosing, through psychotherapy and other methods, I had honed my awareness of emotions and thoughts, interrupted old patterns, and engaged in new behaviors, or at least paused long enough to recognize when old impulses were surfacing. The tools I used were many: a mantra that provides a reliable perch to rest on when I need to pause; the breath—to slow or enliven my nervous system; visualization of positive resources; and self-compassion. These mindfulness tools were my screwdrivers and wrenches, assisting me in reengineering my thinking, feelings, and beliefs—in short, my way of being. After experiencing the sledgehammers of large-dose psychedelic journeys that had broken up the stranglehold of negative beliefs, I became interested in microdosing as a way to fine-tune the application of the information and insights coming into my awareness.

Dr. James Fadiman and Paul Stamets are renowned researchers who have studied psychedelic microdosing for years, and both speak about how Indigenous peoples have long used microdoses of plant medicines as part of their way of being. In fact, all of us who now research and explore psilocybin mushrooms are indebted, specifically, to the Mazatec curandera (healer) María Sabina Magdalena García, who first introduced them to Westerners in 1955. I acknowledge too that we owe a great deal of appreciation, honor, and respect to Indigenous people who have shared their sacraments and processes. I believe it is essential to respect your sourcing of plant medicines and the cultures they come from in a way that does not harm Indigenous traditions, cultivation, or usage.

I chose to write this guide because the integration of experiences from large or small doses of psychedelics, once you're past the fireworks of the big insights and bliss, can be much more than a carnival ride, if you wish it to be. In the post-euphoric emotions after a psychedelic experience, it can seem simple to apply what you've learned. It is not. But the process can be facilitated in skillful ways and with more pleasure.

The insights from a psychedelic experience are the seeds, and the process of germinating those seeds is integration. Germinating seeds is difficult. You must pay close attention to the environment to nurture a sprout strong enough to be able to push through its protective shell and take root in the soil. In the early stages of integration, our psyche resists change. It wants to stay in what is called our *default mode network*. As Michael Pollan writes in his article "The Trip Treatment," the default mode network is thought to be "the physical counterpart of the autobiographical self, or ego." It's a group of interacting brain regions that are theorized to govern reflection, remembering, how you represent yourself, and more. With every experience, the meaning we make is based on the beliefs we have learned through previous experiences; however, we have the opportunity to update these beliefs with each new experience. For instance, if you grew up around harsh criticism, the repeated experience of that dynamic might make you fearful of judgment and cause you to believe others will always judge you. In this case, maybe you have developed shyness around others as one of your default states—a learned behavior that has become automatic. With mindful attention, you can think about your default states and the conditions causing them and decide on different behaviors. It's possible to modify the default mode network so that you aren't limited by default states and can instead be in authentic connection. Young seedlings, like new insights, require extra attention. As the seedling grows into a young plant, its roots become stronger and more resilient. Yet untended plants will wither. These early to middle stages of integration also require a degree of attention, cultivation, and tools that can support that discipline and care. Eventually the plant becomes more mature and needs less tending. Once the insight has been applied with mastery, and you feel you know it and live it as part of you, the insight is more fully integrated.

Integration is a slow, subtle process of transformation, unique to each individual. The steps of integration can include pausing so that the automatic part of you doesn't act first, identifying what you desire to do, being in alignment with your motivation for change, and applying the changes moment to moment.

In his book *Drug Use for Grown-Ups*, Dr. Carl Hart eloquently argues that each human being has a right to pursue consciousness-altering experiences with drugs in the pursuit of happiness, as long as they are taking care of their responsibilities and not harming anyone else. I agree with Dr. Hart. Any tool that helps you become more aware of the shackles of damaging beliefs that impede your happiness should be accessible to all without interference. I encourage you to come out as fully you, to pursue your own happiness by becoming aware of and applying your knowledge of those things you wish to undo and to learn how to do differently.

    We hope this journal invites you into your own time and space, using microdosing as a tool to examine your own perceptions and consciousness and to apply insights from those subtle edges of awareness into the many facets of your life.

—Amy Wong Hope

INTRODUCTION

Many practical guides have been written about psychedelic usage, including Dr. James Fadiman's classic *The Psychedelic Explorer's Guide*. More recently, books like Michelle Janikian's *Your Psilocybin Mushroom Companion* offer detailed and structured information on safely embarking on psychedelic exploration. If you are following the suggestions in these books or other resources, expect some trial and error when figuring out your dose and schedule.

It's up to you to be well informed and to understand any risks associated with your specific circumstances—particularly if you have preexisting medical conditions or use medications that may be contraindicated for psychedelic usage. If you are taking psychiatric medication, consult with your prescriber or a trained medical professional about your microdosing plans. They can help you identify contraindications and advise you as to specific problems or risks of microdosing while pausing any current medications.

Legal implications may also apply. While psychedelics are decriminalized in certain municipalities that allow possession or have reduced policing or penalties for possession, it is still illegal to sell psychedelics.

Microdosing differs from "journey" or macrodosing. It's a practice that does not require disrupting all of the rhythms of your daily life. At the same time, it's important to microdose responsibly. Some people choose to microdose while carrying on with everyday activities, while others will decide that ethically, practically, or professionally they cannot microdose while managing their regular responsibilities. Amy and Shin Yu, for instance, only microdose on nonwork days. We believe it is beneficial to clear away additional demands or obligations and create a protected experience that can allow you to go inward.

There are benefits to interrupting your routines, but you'll want to figure out what you're comfortable doing while your default mode network (see page 15) is at rest. For Shin Yu, driving, grocery shopping, talking to strangers, and dealing with technology are not beneficial tasks for microdosing days. But bringing a new attention to everyday activities like washing dishes or going for a walk can transform these experiences into exercises in mindfulness.

You may find it useful to keep track of your activities on your microdosing days and note anything that you find enjoyable or stressful. Pay attention to your boundaries and honor them—and note how these activities sit with you on integration days. It can be helpful to refer back to setting, place, and time of day, and even details like what you ate, to ensure that you're not overly focused on physical discomfort while microdosing. It can be easy to feel discouraged when trying something new. We suggest you take note of what is or isn't working for you, so you can fine-tune your approach.

If you're reading this book, it's likely you're seeking to be in the driver's seat of your own experience instead of having that experience managed in a clinical setting. Take this as an opportunity to become an expert on your own therapeutic relationship to microdosing. No two people will be the same. To have an optimal experience, you'll want to understand everything you can about the psychedelic you intend to use and its potential risks to you.

While this book is intended to aid in self-directed healing, it is a good idea to develop a support system when you begin opening the mind to the process of awareness through microdosing. Microdosing opens the door to yourself—in potentially intense ways—and you may want to have people around you like a trusted friend or partner who can support you in your journey. A licensed therapist can also aid in integration while giving you a protected space to process in conversation with another person. By taking these safety precautions before you microdose, you may reduce risk and increase safety. (You'll find a list of resources on page 186.)

THE BENEFITS OF MICRODOSING

Microdosing can yield great benefits, but it's not a miracle cure. Through supporting the development of greater self-awareness, microdosing can help you know yourself and how you move through the world. By unscrewing the default mode network just a little bit, you may open up enough space to observe your life with a little less of your internal micromanager and instead approach or cultivate what is pleasurable, interesting, and life-affirming.

Current research reveals that those who microdose psychedelics report some of the benefits explored in this guided journal, including increased creativity, reduction of dysfunctional beliefs, openness, and ability to apply insight. Yet a correlation does not prove that a psychedelic microdose causes these benefits. Research continues to emerge. (You can find a list of recent studies and other research sources in the bibliography on page 184.)

GETTING TO KNOW YOURSELF

Microdosing can provide the opportunity to slow down, feel, and process emotions and sensations that are easily bypassed in our all-too-busy world.

For Amy, trying to make sense of the news of the world while holding a stable anchor of presence with her psychotherapy clients can be a challenge. She is very serious about her self-care routine, and she must have time to process the news on her own so that she can come back to a neutral place in order to be fully present for others.

Being present isn't easy in hard times. We have all indulged in "doom scrolling" or the superficial connections of social media. But these attempts at escape are just that. Being absent from oneself never really helps in the end.

Microdosing is one of the tools that can help in these challenging times. Slowing down, entering into a private ritual, and reorienting to what is important to us are essential to prevent burnout. We are more able to identify which discomforts shouldn't be tolerated or how to tolerate more easily those things we can't change. Paying attention to the body's sensations that signal a "yes" or "no" helps us honor emotions that we might normally bypass. It's a way of being responsible to yourself. Trying to prevent burnout is important, but it happens; and when it does, we must stop, feel, sense, and reflect…and *then* decide. Microdosing is a tool that can facilitate a response instead of a reaction.

Self-reflection, contemplation, and the meaning we choose to make are the only currencies that are fully within our own control. So it's worth it to take the time and make the effort to tune in.

Microdosing doesn't make us do or not do anything. It's an ally to attention—to help us perceive with new eyes, ears, skin…and mind. Its effects have frequently invited us toward an inward attention that guides us in the midst of difficult situations. The result can bring us to a life closer to our authentic self-expression.

Being radically present to one's own feelings and sensations is necessary to live an empowered, embodied life. Microdosing can facilitate this if you choose to use the experience in that way. As you orient yourself to observe and move in ways that are more aligned with your values, you take up space for yourself and know why you're taking up that space. By responding to life as the full, integral you, you might reconnect with other forgotten parts of yourself.

CONNECTING THROUGH RELATIONSHIPS

In the garden, there are plants that coexist as happy neighbors, while others crowd one another. The latter require pruning or relocation. Relationships are not so different, in that certain connections support and energize us while others feel draining or constrain us. Some relationships help you feel spacious and at ease, while others constrict and require you to operate out of alignment with your whole self.

Developmental psychologist Dr. Donald Winnicott theorized that a young infant does not initially know she is a separate entity from her birth parent, but she develops awareness of herself through her caregiver's attention. A parent smiles at her baby, and it indicates to the infant that she exists and is a joy. We all make bids for connection in many ways—a handshake, a smile, a greeting. Responses to these bids connect us to one another.

Similarly, mushrooms reach their mycelial threads through nature, linking separate organisms to one another, sharing information and evolutionary biological support. In his book *Mycelium Running*, renowned mycologist Paul Stamets posits that "mycelium is the neurological network of nature. Interlacing mosaics of mycelium infuse habitats with information-sharing membranes. These membranes are aware, react to change, and collectively have the long-term health of the host environment in mind." Relationships are like mycelial threads between humans. We sense ourselves in different ways in the world when we experience ourselves in connection with others.

This interconnectedness can have benefits but can also pose problems. In her years of working with clients in psychotherapy, Amy has seen firsthand that when people grow up with family relationships that are negative and shaming, they believe they are defective. Sometimes they overcompensate in ways that are not true to themselves, and they experience depression, high anxiety, and burnout.

Since one of the benefits of microdosing is heightened attention to one's own emotions and sensations, it naturally follows that another benefit of microdosing is becoming more conscious of your connections and how they affect you. When there is a healthy connection, there is reciprocity and an energy that flows back and forth. You are magnetized to certain qualities in another person, and they, likewise, are attracted to your unique qualities. Ideally, both sides of this connection equally give and receive. Both sides are energized and supported. The tendrils of who you are entwine with the tendrils of the other—an act of vulnerability. This can offer up a feeling of sweetness and belonging: knowing you exist and matter, knowing you are seen.

When you notice friction and burnout in connection with others, it's an opportunity to decide what's best for you. Knowing your boundaries means you know where you end and the other begins. This is an integral part of any healthy relationship, group, or tribe. Any relationship can have dead leaves and rot that nobody wants to look at. The space between you and the other may feel overly fussy, tense, or rife with interactions that are reactive. When a relationship isn't healthy, start by identifying what you were seeking in the other and honestly assess whether you overcompensated or minimized yourself in pursuit of it.

Microdosing can be an ally to honoring yourself within relationships. Can you track your own emotions and sensations as you are in relationship with the other? Or do you only sense the other person (or group)?

As you sense yourself in your own body and emotions, ask yourself, *Is my focus on my own experience or theirs? Is there a balanced and equal interchange of self and other? Do I limit what I reveal about myself and feel like I must choose my words too carefully, or can I relax and say what's on my mind?* When we fully and vulnerably express ourselves and can feel another receive what we are saying (and vice versa), there is an undeniable ease and satisfaction in the feeling of our whole self meeting another's.

Being in an authentic connection feels like that— a contented sigh, a falling back on a soft bed or fresh-cut grass warmed by the sun, belonging.

EXPLORING YOUR IDENTITY IN THE WORLD

> *To be nobody-but-yourself—in a world which is doing its best, night and day, to make you everybody else—means to fight the hardest battle which any human being can fight.*
>
> —*E. E. Cummings*

Exploring identity is a complex, multidimensional, iterative process. Think about when you meet someone for the first time. Often they ask you what you do or about your background. But your profession or family is just a small fraction of what constitutes your identity. Identity is defined in part by what you consider to be important to your core sense of self. But identity is also imposed upon us through culture, society, systems, laws, family structures, relationships, jobs, and your genetic makeup. All of these factors can cause you to be perceived in ways that are based on biases rather than your own self-definition. Without knowing it, you might find yourself living a conditioned identity that has been entrained and as tightly controlled as the growth of a bonsai tree. But who is the gardener, and did you consent to these forces entraining you?

As you consider your own identity, ask yourself, *What is important to me? Which identities did I choose, and which were imposed upon me? What assumptions do I face every day about who I am?*

The groundbreaking work of BIPOC and social justice scholars and activists has given us language to reexamine the constructs of identities that are marginalized and pathologized within the dominant culture. Many of us have experienced the difficulties of this firsthand. If you are disabled, there are laws to protect you and systems in place to ensure certain accommodations, but socially, culturally, and professionally, you might have been treated differently, overlooked, or considered less able. If you are a woman, you may have experienced sexist assumptions, and your right to bodily autonomy is in question. If you are a parent—especially a primary caregiver—you may have been excluded from opportunities because that work isn't perceived as having value. If you're older than sixty, maybe you've been assumed to be less professionally capable. If you have a Muslim last name, you might have faced unreasonable extra scrutiny at security checks. And if you have an identity that has been minoritized due to your racial or ethnic background, there are myriad ways in which you may have had to live with or dispel assumptions, biases, and prejudices.

Recognizing biases and naming them is exhausting. Trying to live authentically, to not be in perpetual reaction to biases, is a never-ending challenge. Many people move through the world in a state of hypervigilance or suffer under the strain of these biases in their relationships.

In the days following a recent microdose, Amy was struck by the small doses of awareness that surfaced as she moved through her world. There were more instances where she stopped, paused, and took time to pay attention, reflect, and honor what was arising. In that reflection space, the small doses of awareness and meaning-making became a helpful way to iterate and reevaluate her questions about identity. Examining and forming your identity, by yourself and in relation to others, is a continual process. We constantly seek nourishment, connection, and actualization. We are the plant reaching its roots for water, the mushroom spreading its mycelium in adaptation.

Microdosing as a conduit of awareness can help navigate the edges of where you meet the world. Remember, it's not the psychedelic microdose that makes the change. It's your commitment to you. Your awareness and your identity minister to and transform you through integration, to help you arrive at an authentic self.

GETTING CONNECTED TO CREATIVITY

One of Shin Yu's biggest hesitations about psychedelics was her anxiety about how they might change her connectedness to creativity. She'd spent more than a decade on and off prescription medications trying to manage lifelong depression. And over those periods of being medicated, she found the drugs could blunt emotions and cut off access to a complex inner terrain that often enriched her life and work as a writer. A person does not have to suffer to make great art, but the creative muse can be fickle and unpredictable. As a person who values creativity, she didn't want to risk losing any parts of herself for fear that she might not be able to write again.

In her book *A Really Good Day*, Ayelet Waldman considered the possibilities of combining microdosing with a creative practice. Waldman's book traced the impact of her experiences with LSD over a month, during which she saw dramatic changes in her overall mindset. As for writing, she had very productive writing days and not-so-productive writing days—*just like writers who aren't microdosing*. What microdosing did do for Waldman was to help her relax into seeing her own mind more clearly without judgment. If the mind is feeling quick to judge, curiosity can't come forward.

It's not just artists who choose psychedelics as a way to connect to their minds in new ways. People working in many other spaces have turned to microdosing to inspire innovative thinking and improve focus. Justin Zhu, cofounder of the tech start-up Iterable, has spoken about how his journey with LSD helped him pivot from being a tech executive to directing his energies toward activism. He took the focus and personal insights that microdosing revealed to him and cofounded Stand with Asian Americans, an organization that mobilizes Asian American business leaders in fighting violence against their community.

Working with LSD allowed Zhu to get in touch with a deeper sense of self and to connect to his authentic voice. This was particularly profound in a moment when our nation saw a huge uptick in violent crimes against Asian Americans. He developed a deeper appreciation of the complexity of his parents' immigrant experience and began to consider how he could better center his personal and cultural values in his work. Creative thinking resulted in his opening up to new possibilities and ways of being.

Creativity isn't just about the end goal of writing a book, chiseling away at a chunk of marble, or sculpting molten glass. The muscle we want to work is creative thinking itself, strengthening our connection to the creative spirit, which is the same place from which we might cook an inspired meal, plant a backyard pollinator garden, or spend an afternoon playing with our inner or actual child.

To encourage creativity and an awareness of your inner states, try the reflective questions in this journal to inspire your own thinking and writing. These prompts might seem simple, but they are an invitation to relate to yourself without the constant story of your life humming in the background. Creativity is the opportunity to reclaim parts of yourself by rewriting the narrative that you've been told about yourself, to arrive at your own essential questions and truths.

WEEK ONE

CREATING SAFETY

Psychedelics are a popular and growing trend in therapeutic and creative communities. It seems as if everyone, from suburban parents to CEOs, is exploring the mental health benefits associated with microdosing.

Before microdosing, examine your purpose. Maybe you have taken larger therapeutic doses of psychedelics and are interested in a more subtle experience of observing your mind. Perhaps you're curious about the power of plant medicines to treat depression, facilitate personal growth, or heal past traumas. Whatever brings you to this moment, it's helpful as a self-guided learner to get in touch with your hopes, expectations, and goals.

Microdosing can open new awareness and renewed focus by providing you with different opportunities to connect to your mind, but if you have experienced depression for most of your life, it may not be realistic to expect depression to vanish after microdosing one time, or even many times. Like a stalagmite formation, depression builds up in layers over time. If your goal is to calm your daily anxieties, your experiences while microdosing may give you useful information about specific activities that induce stress, but microdosing won't make deeply ingrained habits and patterns disappear.

What are you asking of this journey right now? Make a list of what you want to gain from or experience when microdosing. Which of these expectations seem most realistic?

After you've explored your inner state, take some time to think about what you need to set the stage for a comfortable experience. When we get ready to go to sleep, we close the blinds to block out the light. We put away our devices and silence cell phone alerts. We may close the door to minimize noise or warm the bedroom. Consider the routines you need to create a safe and positive microdosing experience. Often circumstances aren't ideal, or life demands our attention, but what basic conditions must be met for you to open into the experience of microdosing?

INQUIRIES

What do you hope to learn about yourself
or experience through microdosing?

What are you seeking to explore or heal?
Why is this important to you right now?

What kind of microdosing ritual can
you create that will allow you to slow down
and pay attention to your experiences?

What kind of mini refuge or retreat do you want
to create for your microdosing days?

What intention will help you maintain your
focus on microdosing days?

What do you plan to do or not do with what
you become aware of?

INSIGHTS AND OBSERVATIONS

DATE:

MY OVERALL MOOD IS:
- ◯ Neutral
- ◯ Curious
- ◯ Irritated
- ◯ Calm
- ◯ Worried
- ◯ Excited
- ◯ Burnt Out
- ◯ Preoccupied
- ◯ Contemplative
- ◯ Other:

THE EMOTIONS I FEEL TODAY ARE:
- ◯ Happiness
- ◯ Frustration
- ◯ Sadness
- ◯ Anger
- ◯ Peace
- ◯ Apathy
- ◯ Overwhelm
- ◯ Other:

MY BODY FEELS:
- ◯ Heavy
- ◯ Light
- ◯ Relaxed
- ◯ Alert
- ◯ Grounded
- ◯ Energized
- ◯ Constricted
- ◯ Agitated
- ◯ Other:

WHAT DO I WANT TO CONTINUE NOTICING OR DOING?

WHAT INSIGHTS AND OBSERVATIONS DO I WANT TO COME BACK TO?

INSIGHTS AND OBSERVATIONS

DATE:

MY OVERALL MOOD IS:
- ○ Neutral
- ○ Curious
- ○ Irritated
- ○ Calm
- ○ Worried
- ○ Excited
- ○ Burnt Out
- ○ Preoccupied
- ○ Contemplative
- ○ Other:

THE EMOTIONS I FEEL TODAY ARE:
- ○ Happiness
- ○ Frustration
- ○ Sadness
- ○ Anger
- ○ Peace
- ○ Apathy
- ○ Overwhelm
- ○ Other:

MY BODY FEELS:
- ○ Heavy
- ○ Light
- ○ Relaxed
- ○ Alert
- ○ Grounded
- ○ Energized
- ○ Constricted
- ○ Agitated
- ○ Other:

WHAT DO I WANT TO CONTINUE NOTICING OR DOING?

WHAT INSIGHTS AND OBSERVATIONS DO I WANT TO COME BACK TO?

INSIGHTS AND OBSERVATIONS

DATE:

MY OVERALL MOOD IS:
- ○ Neutral
- ○ Curious
- ○ Irritated
- ○ Calm
- ○ Worried
- ○ Excited
- ○ Burnt Out
- ○ Preoccupied
- ○ Contemplative
- ○ Other: _____

THE EMOTIONS I FEEL TODAY ARE:
- ○ Happiness
- ○ Frustration
- ○ Sadness
- ○ Anger
- ○ Peace
- ○ Apathy
- ○ Overwhelm
- ○ Other: _____

MY BODY FEELS:
- ○ Heavy
- ○ Light
- ○ Relaxed
- ○ Alert
- ○ Grounded
- ○ Energized
- ○ Constricted
- ○ Agitated
- ○ Other: _____

WHAT DO I WANT TO CONTINUE NOTICING OR DOING?

WHAT INSIGHTS AND OBSERVATIONS DO I WANT TO COME BACK TO?

INSIGHTS AND OBSERVATIONS

DATE:

MY OVERALL MOOD IS:
- ○ Neutral
- ○ Curious
- ○ Irritated
- ○ Calm
- ○ Worried
- ○ Excited
- ○ Burnt Out
- ○ Preoccupied
- ○ Contemplative
- ○ Other:

THE EMOTIONS I FEEL TODAY ARE:
- ○ Happiness
- ○ Frustration
- ○ Sadness
- ○ Anger
- ○ Peace
- ○ Apathy
- ○ Overwhelm
- ○ Other:

MY BODY FEELS:
- ○ Heavy
- ○ Light
- ○ Relaxed
- ○ Alert
- ○ Grounded
- ○ Energized
- ○ Constricted
- ○ Agitated
- ○ Other:

WHAT DO I WANT TO CONTINUE NOTICING OR DOING?

WHAT INSIGHTS AND OBSERVATIONS DO I WANT TO COME BACK TO?

INSIGHTS AND OBSERVATIONS

DATE:

MY OVERALL MOOD IS:
- ○ Neutral
- ○ Curious
- ○ Irritated
- ○ Calm
- ○ Worried
- ○ Excited
- ○ Burnt Out
- ○ Preoccupied
- ○ Contemplative
- ○ Other:

THE EMOTIONS I FEEL TODAY ARE:
- ○ Happiness
- ○ Frustration
- ○ Sadness
- ○ Anger
- ○ Peace
- ○ Apathy
- ○ Overwhelm
- ○ Other:

MY BODY FEELS:
- ○ Heavy
- ○ Light
- ○ Relaxed
- ○ Alert
- ○ Grounded
- ○ Energized
- ○ Constricted
- ○ Agitated
- ○ Other:

WHAT DO I WANT TO CONTINUE NOTICING OR DOING?

WHAT INSIGHTS AND OBSERVATIONS DO I WANT TO COME BACK TO?

WEEK TWO

LEANING INTO THE SENSES

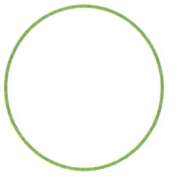ur five senses serve as antennae that help us create our inner landscape. This week, you'll focus on exploring the five senses—sight, sound, taste, touch, and smell—and how they can give you valuable information about how you experience the world.

Technology and nonstop news have made our experience of our surroundings increasingly complex. It's often hard to notice our senses when we are constantly overstimulated. And it's rare that our eyes or ears or mind get a break long enough to pay deep attention.

How can we use microdosing as a tool to reset and reorient ourselves to our five senses? Whether on an integration day or a day that you've planned to microdose, you might try creating a ritual of sensory experiences for yourself.

Light a stick of incense, and notice the various notes of fragrance. What does the incense smell like before it's lit? What spices and qualities come forward when the incense burns? How does it smell once it's extinguished? Imagine the journey the incense went through before entering your home. Indian sandalwood is revered for its ability to help focus and relax the mind during meditation. A sandalwood tree doesn't reach maturity for sixty to eighty years.

Decades of sun and rain nourish the trees that provide the material for one small stick of incense. Consider the labor involved in harvesting and preparing the wood for production. When we experience incense with all of our senses, we can grow our awareness and appreciation of our beautiful world.

Get in touch with gentle activities that allow you to fully sink into all of your senses. Consider how our senses come alive in relationship to nature. In your garden, stir up some soil with your bare hands. Plant a seed and water it. As the plant grows and thrives, you nurture your relationship to nature, and the earth gives back to you.

The natural world can invite us to focus our attention on the scent of fresh herbs, like lavender, or on the sweetness of a raspberry plucked straight off the vine. Nature wraps us in the pleasure of our own senses. In this space, we can be at ease. We can remember what it feels like to slow down and be present with our experiences. And this can allow us to reset throughout the chaos of a busy day.

Where do your senses take you? Try taking a deeper dive into two of your five senses to notice where you choose to direct them. Observe where they take you from moment to moment.

INQUIRIES

Take a few moments to let your gaze wander and write down everything you notice around you.

Pick an essential oil or kitchen herb. Identify the type of plant it comes from. Breathe in deeply. What thoughts or emotions do you associate with this scent? How does this scent activate or calm you?

Take a shower and notice how it feels when the water contacts your skin. How do you connect to your own body and pleasure?

Hold a piece of fruit. Examine its color and texture, and explore what it feels like in your hand. Smell it. Bite it. Chew it. Which tastes do you prefer, and why?

Find a quiet space. What sounds catch your attention? What do you notice about them?

Which senses dominate your awareness, and which require you to shift your attention to experience them more fully?

INSIGHTS AND OBSERVATIONS

DATE:

MY OVERALL MOOD IS:

- ○ Neutral
- ○ Curious
- ○ Irritated
- ○ Calm
- ○ Worried
- ○ Excited
- ○ Burnt Out
- ○ Preoccupied
- ○ Contemplative
- ○ Other: _____

THE EMOTIONS I FEEL TODAY ARE:

- ○ Happiness
- ○ Frustration
- ○ Sadness
- ○ Anger
- ○ Peace
- ○ Apathy
- ○ Overwhelm
- ○ Other: _____

MY BODY FEELS:

- ○ Heavy
- ○ Light
- ○ Relaxed
- ○ Alert
- ○ Grounded
- ○ Energized
- ○ Constricted
- ○ Agitated
- ○ Other: _____

WHAT DO I WANT TO CONTINUE NOTICING OR DOING?

WHAT INSIGHTS AND OBSERVATIONS DO I WANT TO COME BACK TO?

INSIGHTS AND OBSERVATIONS

DATE:

MY OVERALL MOOD IS:

- ○ Neutral
- ○ Curious
- ○ Irritated
- ○ Calm
- ○ Worried
- ○ Excited
- ○ Burnt Out
- ○ Preoccupied
- ○ Contemplative
- ○ Other:

THE EMOTIONS I FEEL TODAY ARE:

- ○ Happiness
- ○ Frustration
- ○ Sadness
- ○ Anger
- ○ Peace
- ○ Apathy
- ○ Overwhelm
- ○ Other: _____

MY BODY FEELS:

- ○ Heavy
- ○ Light
- ○ Relaxed
- ○ Alert
- ○ Grounded
- ○ Energized
- ○ Constricted
- ○ Agitated
- ○ Other:

WHAT DO I WANT TO CONTINUE NOTICING OR DOING?

WHAT INSIGHTS AND OBSERVATIONS DO I WANT TO COME BACK TO?

INSIGHTS AND OBSERVATIONS

DATE:

MY OVERALL MOOD IS:

- ◯ Neutral
- ◯ Curious
- ◯ Irritated
- ◯ Calm
- ◯ Worried
- ◯ Excited
- ◯ Burnt Out
- ◯ Preoccupied
- ◯ Contemplative
- ◯ Other:

THE EMOTIONS I FEEL TODAY ARE:

- ◯ Happiness
- ◯ Frustration
- ◯ Sadness
- ◯ Anger
- ◯ Peace
- ◯ Apathy
- ◯ Overwhelm
- ◯ Other:

MY BODY FEELS:

- ◯ Heavy
- ◯ Light
- ◯ Relaxed
- ◯ Alert
- ◯ Grounded
- ◯ Energized
- ◯ Constricted
- ◯ Agitated
- ◯ Other:

WHAT DO I WANT TO CONTINUE NOTICING OR DOING?

WHAT INSIGHTS AND OBSERVATIONS DO I WANT TO COME BACK TO?

INSIGHTS AND OBSERVATIONS

DATE:

MY OVERALL MOOD IS:

- ○ Neutral
- ○ Curious
- ○ Irritated
- ○ Calm
- ○ Worried
- ○ Excited
- ○ Burnt Out
- ○ Preoccupied
- ○ Contemplative
- ○ Other:

THE EMOTIONS I FEEL TODAY ARE:

- ○ Happiness
- ○ Frustration
- ○ Sadness
- ○ Anger
- ○ Peace
- ○ Apathy
- ○ Overwhelm
- ○ Other:

MY BODY FEELS:

- ○ Heavy
- ○ Light
- ○ Relaxed
- ○ Alert
- ○ Grounded
- ○ Energized
- ○ Constricted
- ○ Agitated
- ○ Other:

WHAT DO I WANT TO CONTINUE NOTICING OR DOING?

WHAT INSIGHTS AND OBSERVATIONS DO I WANT TO COME BACK TO?

INSIGHTS AND OBSERVATIONS

DATE:

MY OVERALL MOOD IS:

- ◯ Neutral
- ◯ Curious
- ◯ Irritated
- ◯ Calm
- ◯ Worried
- ◯ Excited
- ◯ Burnt Out
- ◯ Preoccupied
- ◯ Contemplative
- ◯ Other:

THE EMOTIONS I FEEL TODAY ARE:

- ◯ Happiness
- ◯ Frustration
- ◯ Sadness
- ◯ Anger
- ◯ Peace
- ◯ Apathy
- ◯ Overwhelm
- ◯ Other:

MY BODY FEELS:

- ◯ Heavy
- ◯ Light
- ◯ Relaxed
- ◯ Alert
- ◯ Grounded
- ◯ Energized
- ◯ Constricted
- ◯ Agitated
- ◯ Other:

WHAT DO I WANT TO CONTINUE NOTICING OR DOING?

WHAT INSIGHTS AND OBSERVATIONS DO I WANT TO COME BACK TO?

WEEK THREE

HOW I SEE ME

For many of us in our unsure teen years, the mirror is a constant companion, a distorted reflection in which we contemplate flaws and how to hide them. But as we mature and pursue a more authentic relationship with ourselves, we want to be comfortable with our physical bodies and our presentation in the world.

After a recent microdose, Amy studied herself in a mirror—the way her eyes moved, the texture of her skin and hair, the shape of her lips—and practiced being present with how she saw herself in that moment. What she saw made her realize that being radically present allows us to truly see ourselves. No matter who we are or what we look like, our culture constantly manipulates our self-perception, imposing subconscious expectations to get us to buy something or work harder for someone else. It is only by being radically present to ourselves in full honesty that we can avoid being manipulated by artifice.

Try standing in front of a mirror after bathing. Take your time, and don't get pulled into getting ready for your day. Gaze into your eyes. Take in the textures of your hair, skin, and body. Notice the thoughts and emotions that arise. If there is judgment, label it as judgment. Go back to observing yourself in the mirror. Notice the shapes of your face, hair, and body. Notice how you move. Take in your image and try to look beyond what you see. Try to identify what's underneath your physical appearance. Reclaim your one-on-one relationship with yourself.

Only you know if you're being honest with yourself. Many times the mirror has been a place where we've noticed and questioned whether we're being honest with ourselves. Other times, it is a place where we can come to honestly appreciate ourselves as we are. The recognition that mirror-gazing can bring isn't about physical appearance. It can be an entry point to reckoning with underlying emotions and a place to reflect on your identity. When you look clearly at yourself in the present, and then beyond that initial reflected image, what do you see?

Roles, relationships, and careers *can* be a mirror. And like a mirror, they can be healthy or unhealthy. How do you see yourself today based on these mirrors? How much of what you see reflects the real you?

What you do day to day, how you live from moment to moment, is a mirror too. What do you do with what you become aware of?

Keep asking yourself, *How do I see me?*

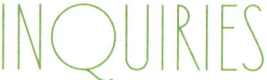

INQUIRIES

What defines how you see yourself?

What do you celebrate in what you see?

What do you hide or dislike or consider imperfect? How can you embrace and accept these things?

What parts of yourself are you curious to explore and give space to? How will you explore these parts of yourself?

INSIGHTS AND OBSERVATIONS

DATE:

MY OVERALL MOOD IS:

- ○ Neutral
- ○ Curious
- ○ Irritated
- ○ Calm
- ○ Worried
- ○ Excited
- ○ Burnt Out
- ○ Preoccupied
- ○ Contemplative
- ○ Other:

THE EMOTIONS I FEEL TODAY ARE:

- ○ Happiness
- ○ Frustration
- ○ Sadness
- ○ Anger
- ○ Peace
- ○ Apathy
- ○ Overwhelm
- ○ Other:

MY BODY FEELS:

- ○ Heavy
- ○ Light
- ○ Relaxed
- ○ Alert
- ○ Grounded
- ○ Energized
- ○ Constricted
- ○ Agitated
- ○ Other:

WHAT DO I WANT TO CONTINUE NOTICING OR DOING?

WHAT INSIGHTS AND OBSERVATIONS DO I WANT TO COME BACK TO?

INSIGHTS AND OBSERVATIONS

DATE:

MY OVERALL MOOD IS:

- ○ Neutral
- ○ Curious
- ○ Irritated
- ○ Calm
- ○ Worried
- ○ Excited
- ○ Burnt Out
- ○ Preoccupied
- ○ Contemplative
- ○ Other:

THE EMOTIONS I FEEL TODAY ARE:

- ○ Happiness
- ○ Frustration
- ○ Sadness
- ○ Anger
- ○ Peace
- ○ Apathy
- ○ Overwhelm
- ○ Other:

MY BODY FEELS:

- ○ Heavy
- ○ Light
- ○ Relaxed
- ○ Alert
- ○ Grounded
- ○ Energized
- ○ Constricted
- ○ Agitated
- ○ Other:

WHAT DO I WANT TO CONTINUE NOTICING OR DOING?

WHAT INSIGHTS AND OBSERVATIONS DO I WANT TO COME BACK TO?

INSIGHTS AND OBSERVATIONS

DATE:

MY OVERALL MOOD IS:
- ◯ Neutral
- ◯ Curious
- ◯ Irritated
- ◯ Calm
- ◯ Worried
- ◯ Excited
- ◯ Burnt Out
- ◯ Preoccupied
- ◯ Contemplative
- ◯ Other:

THE EMOTIONS I FEEL TODAY ARE:
- ◯ Happiness
- ◯ Frustration
- ◯ Sadness
- ◯ Anger
- ◯ Peace
- ◯ Apathy
- ◯ Overwhelm
- ◯ Other:

MY BODY FEELS:
- ◯ Heavy
- ◯ Light
- ◯ Relaxed
- ◯ Alert
- ◯ Grounded
- ◯ Energized
- ◯ Constricted
- ◯ Agitated
- ◯ Other:

WHAT DO I WANT TO CONTINUE NOTICING OR DOING?

WHAT INSIGHTS AND OBSERVATIONS DO I WANT TO COME BACK TO?

INSIGHTS AND OBSERVATIONS

DATE:

MY OVERALL MOOD IS:

- ○ Neutral
- ○ Curious
- ○ Irritated
- ○ Calm
- ○ Worried
- ○ Excited
- ○ Burnt Out
- ○ Preoccupied
- ○ Contemplative
- ○ Other: _____

THE EMOTIONS I FEEL TODAY ARE:

- ○ Happiness
- ○ Frustration
- ○ Sadness
- ○ Anger
- ○ Peace
- ○ Apathy
- ○ Overwhelm
- ○ Other: _____

MY BODY FEELS:

- ○ Heavy
- ○ Light
- ○ Relaxed
- ○ Alert
- ○ Grounded
- ○ Energized
- ○ Constricted
- ○ Agitated
- ○ Other: _____

WHAT DO I WANT TO CONTINUE NOTICING OR DOING?

WHAT INSIGHTS AND OBSERVATIONS DO I WANT TO COME BACK TO?

INSIGHTS AND OBSERVATIONS

DATE:

MY OVERALL MOOD IS:
- ○ Neutral
- ○ Curious
- ○ Irritated
- ○ Calm
- ○ Worried
- ○ Excited
- ○ Burnt Out
- ○ Preoccupied
- ○ Contemplative
- ○ Other:

THE EMOTIONS I FEEL TODAY ARE:
- ○ Happiness
- ○ Frustration
- ○ Sadness
- ○ Anger
- ○ Peace
- ○ Apathy
- ○ Overwhelm
- ○ Other:

MY BODY FEELS:
- ○ Heavy
- ○ Light
- ○ Relaxed
- ○ Alert
- ○ Grounded
- ○ Energized
- ○ Constricted
- ○ Agitated
- ○ Other:

WHAT DO I WANT TO CONTINUE NOTICING OR DOING?

WHAT INSIGHTS AND OBSERVATIONS DO I WANT TO COME BACK TO?

WEEK FOUR

HOW I CONNECT WITH THE WORLD

When you arrive in a new place, consider the worlds you've left and the worlds you're entering. These are opportunities to step outside your habitual identities and see yourself in a new light. You may learn that how you see yourself differs from how others view or experience you.

Consider all that you are becoming aware of on your microdosing journey. Is how you see yourself aligned with how others view you? Your observations and what you do with that information provide an opportunity to better articulate who you are and what's important to you.

Shin Yu grew up in a multiracial community on the West Coast. In Southern California, she fit into a melting pot of black and brown families where being the kid of immigrants was commonplace. But as an adult living and working in places like Arkansas and Texas, she was viewed primarily through the lens of her race and gender. She was perceived as either a pushover or a dragon lady—or somehow both. But the way in which she really wanted her colleagues to see her was as the artist, teacher, and leader she was.

When Amy's parents sent her on a cultural tour to reconnect to her Chinese roots, she realized how different she was from her peers on the trip, all of whom were Chinese American like her. Amy grew up outside the larger

Boston Chinese community on Cape Cod, where she'd been one of only three Asians in her school. She didn't grow up speaking or understanding Cantonese, but most of the other teens on her tour did.

The local Chinese people understood that Amy was born in the United States and had not been exposed to the language, and they were kind and empathetic—they made an effort to connect. In contrast, the kids on Amy's tour excluded her and another monolingual student. This experience gave Amy valuable perspective on how she wanted to make inclusive spaces for those with a range of cultural and linguistic identities.

Both Amy and Shin Yu had to examine their own identities based on how others saw and treated them. Each had moments of reckoning that involved finding ways to connect to the cultures in which they found themselves while staying true to their own identities.

Consider a time when you've had to step outside your comfort zone and into a new environment. Maybe you relocated to a new country or city. Or maybe you changed jobs or left one industry for another. Consider your existing worlds. Who are you within these worlds, and how do you connect to them? What have your peers assumed about you? How do their perceptions align or misalign with who you are?

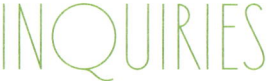

What are people surprised to learn about you?

What do you wish people knew about you?

What prevents you from sharing these parts of yourself? What do you gain or lose by withholding these parts?

When you meet a new person, how do you assume they see you? What do you hope they see? What do you hide?

How are you aligned with your vision of your identity and what others see in you? If there is misalignment, what does that mean to you? How do you wish to meet the world?

INSIGHTS AND OBSERVATIONS

DATE:

MY OVERALL MOOD IS:

- ○ Neutral
- ○ Curious
- ○ Irritated
- ○ Calm
- ○ Worried
- ○ Excited
- ○ Burnt Out
- ○ Preoccupied
- ○ Contemplative
- ○ Other:

THE EMOTIONS I FEEL TODAY ARE:

- ○ Happiness
- ○ Frustration
- ○ Sadness
- ○ Anger
- ○ Peace
- ○ Apathy
- ○ Overwhelm
- ○ Other:

MY BODY FEELS:

- ○ Heavy
- ○ Light
- ○ Relaxed
- ○ Alert
- ○ Grounded
- ○ Energized
- ○ Constricted
- ○ Agitated
- ○ Other:

WHAT DO I WANT TO CONTINUE NOTICING OR DOING?

WHAT INSIGHTS AND OBSERVATIONS DO I WANT TO COME BACK TO?

INSIGHTS AND OBSERVATIONS

DATE:

MY OVERALL MOOD IS:
- ○ Neutral
- ○ Curious
- ○ Irritated
- ○ Calm
- ○ Worried
- ○ Excited
- ○ Burnt Out
- ○ Preoccupied
- ○ Contemplative
- ○ Other:

THE EMOTIONS I FEEL TODAY ARE:
- ○ Happiness
- ○ Frustration
- ○ Sadness
- ○ Anger
- ○ Peace
- ○ Apathy
- ○ Overwhelm
- ○ Other:

MY BODY FEELS:
- ○ Heavy
- ○ Light
- ○ Relaxed
- ○ Alert
- ○ Grounded
- ○ Energized
- ○ Constricted
- ○ Agitated
- ○ Other:

WHAT DO I WANT TO CONTINUE NOTICING OR DOING?

WHAT INSIGHTS AND OBSERVATIONS DO I WANT TO COME BACK TO?

INSIGHTS AND OBSERVATIONS

DATE:

MY OVERALL MOOD IS:
- ○ Neutral
- ○ Curious
- ○ Irritated
- ○ Calm
- ○ Worried
- ○ Excited
- ○ Burnt Out
- ○ Preoccupied
- ○ Contemplative
- ○ Other:

THE EMOTIONS I FEEL TODAY ARE:
- ○ Happiness
- ○ Frustration
- ○ Sadness
- ○ Anger
- ○ Peace
- ○ Apathy
- ○ Overwhelm
- ○ Other:

MY BODY FEELS:
- ○ Heavy
- ○ Light
- ○ Relaxed
- ○ Alert
- ○ Grounded
- ○ Energized
- ○ Constricted
- ○ Agitated
- ○ Other:

WHAT DO I WANT TO CONTINUE NOTICING OR DOING?

WHAT INSIGHTS AND OBSERVATIONS DO I WANT TO COME BACK TO?

INSIGHTS AND OBSERVATIONS

DATE:

MY OVERALL MOOD IS:

- ○ Neutral
- ○ Curious
- ○ Irritated
- ○ Calm
- ○ Worried
- ○ Excited
- ○ Burnt Out
- ○ Preoccupied
- ○ Contemplative
- ○ Other:

THE EMOTIONS I FEEL TODAY ARE:

- ○ Happiness
- ○ Frustration
- ○ Sadness
- ○ Anger
- ○ Peace
- ○ Apathy
- ○ Overwhelm
- ○ Other:

MY BODY FEELS:

- ○ Heavy
- ○ Light
- ○ Relaxed
- ○ Alert
- ○ Grounded
- ○ Energized
- ○ Constricted
- ○ Agitated
- ○ Other:

WHAT DO I WANT TO CONTINUE NOTICING OR DOING?

WHAT INSIGHTS AND OBSERVATIONS DO I WANT TO COME BACK TO?

INSIGHTS AND OBSERVATIONS

DATE:

MY OVERALL MOOD IS:

- ◯ Neutral
- ◯ Curious
- ◯ Irritated
- ◯ Calm
- ◯ Worried
- ◯ Excited
- ◯ Burnt Out
- ◯ Preoccupied
- ◯ Contemplative
- ◯ Other:

THE EMOTIONS I FEEL TODAY ARE:

- ◯ Happiness
- ◯ Frustration
- ◯ Sadness
- ◯ Anger
- ◯ Peace
- ◯ Apathy
- ◯ Overwhelm
- ◯ Other:

MY BODY FEELS:

- ◯ Heavy
- ◯ Light
- ◯ Relaxed
- ◯ Alert
- ◯ Grounded
- ◯ Energized
- ◯ Constricted
- ◯ Agitated
- ◯ Other:

WHAT DO I WANT TO CONTINUE NOTICING OR DOING?

WHAT INSIGHTS AND OBSERVATIONS DO I WANT TO COME BACK TO?

WEEK FIVE

WHAT I'VE ASSUMED TO BE TRUE

Social conditioning affects the way we regard others when it comes to gender, class, size, age, and other characteristics. But more than that, it affects how we see *ourselves* and places limits on our own capacities for growth. We may prevent ourselves from evolving into bigger, more fulfilled versions of ourselves when we are held back by self-limiting beliefs.

Microdosing has helped Shin Yu differentiate her values and experiences from those of her family of origin. Shin Yu's parents immigrated to the United States with hopes of achieving the American dream: a house, a family, a fulfilling career, and financial well-being. For them, these markers would prove that they belonged. But instead, her parents fell deep into debt and suffered in jobs where their talents weren't recognized or honored. They raised children who struggled to find their place, caught between two cultures.

But despite their experiences, Shin Yu's parents still believed in the American dream for her. They saw her life as an extension of their own, and she learned from them how to be a good, hardworking Asian daughter. Buying into their belief system made it hard to move on when she first confronted difficulty in the workplace. Unhealthy professional environments took the place of an unhealthy family environment and normalized harmful dynamics.

The clarity gained through microdosing helped Shin Yu realize that her identity extended beyond a toxic workplace and beyond her family's expectations. She could choose a dream of her own. With each microdosing experience, Shin Yu found a new opportunity to relate to her own mind, emotions, and needs, which were distinct from the systems that dominated her early life.

Look and listen. You may be able to finally hear your own voice in the crowd. Keep nurturing that whisper until it's a roar.

In what ways are your own values out of alignment with what you've been socialized or taught to accept as normal?

INQUIRIES

How has living within the body that you were born with affected you as you move through the world?

How do you distinguish between "who I am" and "what I do"?

How has your family of origin informed who you are? What lessons did you learn that empowered or limited you?

What has your socioeconomic status made you believe about your worth?

How has your gender identity helped or hindered how you wish to be and what you wish to do in the world?

What expectations do you continue to meet that have felt constricting, suppressing, too rigid, or too loose?

INSIGHTS AND OBSERVATIONS

DATE:

MY OVERALL MOOD IS:
- ○ Neutral
- ○ Curious
- ○ Irritated
- ○ Calm
- ○ Worried
- ○ Excited
- ○ Burnt Out
- ○ Preoccupied
- ○ Contemplative
- ○ Other:

THE EMOTIONS I FEEL TODAY ARE:
- ○ Happiness
- ○ Frustration
- ○ Sadness
- ○ Anger
- ○ Peace
- ○ Apathy
- ○ Overwhelm
- ○ Other:

MY BODY FEELS:
- ○ Heavy
- ○ Light
- ○ Relaxed
- ○ Alert
- ○ Grounded
- ○ Energized
- ○ Constricted
- ○ Agitated
- ○ Other:

WHAT DO I WANT TO CONTINUE NOTICING OR DOING?

WHAT INSIGHTS AND OBSERVATIONS DO I WANT TO COME BACK TO?

INSIGHTS AND OBSERVATIONS

DATE:

MY OVERALL MOOD IS:

- ○ Neutral
- ○ Curious
- ○ Irritated
- ○ Calm
- ○ Worried
- ○ Excited
- ○ Burnt Out
- ○ Preoccupied
- ○ Contemplative
- ○ Other:

THE EMOTIONS I FEEL TODAY ARE:

- ○ Happiness
- ○ Frustration
- ○ Sadness
- ○ Anger
- ○ Peace
- ○ Apathy
- ○ Overwhelm
- ○ Other:

MY BODY FEELS:

- ○ Heavy
- ○ Light
- ○ Relaxed
- ○ Alert
- ○ Grounded
- ○ Energized
- ○ Constricted
- ○ Agitated
- ○ Other:

WHAT DO I WANT TO CONTINUE NOTICING OR DOING?

WHAT INSIGHTS AND OBSERVATIONS DO I WANT TO COME BACK TO?

INSIGHTS AND OBSERVATIONS

DATE:

MY OVERALL MOOD IS:

- ○ Neutral
- ○ Curious
- ○ Irritated
- ○ Calm
- ○ Worried
- ○ Excited
- ○ Burnt Out
- ○ Preoccupied
- ○ Contemplative
- ○ Other:

THE EMOTIONS I FEEL TODAY ARE:

- ○ Happiness
- ○ Frustration
- ○ Sadness
- ○ Anger
- ○ Peace
- ○ Apathy
- ○ Overwhelm
- ○ Other:

MY BODY FEELS:

- ○ Heavy
- ○ Light
- ○ Relaxed
- ○ Alert
- ○ Grounded
- ○ Energized
- ○ Constricted
- ○ Agitated
- ○ Other:

WHAT DO I WANT TO CONTINUE NOTICING OR DOING?

WHAT INSIGHTS AND OBSERVATIONS DO I WANT TO COME BACK TO?

INSIGHTS AND OBSERVATIONS

DATE:

MY OVERALL MOOD IS:
- ○ Neutral
- ○ Curious
- ○ Irritated
- ○ Calm
- ○ Worried
- ○ Excited
- ○ Burnt Out
- ○ Preoccupied
- ○ Contemplative
- ○ Other:

THE EMOTIONS I FEEL TODAY ARE:
- ○ Happiness
- ○ Frustration
- ○ Sadness
- ○ Anger
- ○ Peace
- ○ Apathy
- ○ Overwhelm
- ○ Other:

MY BODY FEELS:
- ○ Heavy
- ○ Light
- ○ Relaxed
- ○ Alert
- ○ Grounded
- ○ Energized
- ○ Constricted
- ○ Agitated
- ○ Other:

WHAT DO I WANT TO CONTINUE NOTICING OR DOING?

WHAT INSIGHTS AND OBSERVATIONS DO I WANT TO COME BACK TO?

INSIGHTS AND OBSERVATIONS

DATE:

MY OVERALL MOOD IS:

- ○ Neutral
- ○ Curious
- ○ Irritated
- ○ Calm
- ○ Worried
- ○ Excited
- ○ Burnt Out
- ○ Preoccupied
- ○ Contemplative
- ○ Other:

THE EMOTIONS I FEEL TODAY ARE:

- ○ Happiness
- ○ Frustration
- ○ Sadness
- ○ Anger
- ○ Peace
- ○ Apathy
- ○ Overwhelm
- ○ Other:

MY BODY FEELS:

- ○ Heavy
- ○ Light
- ○ Relaxed
- ○ Alert
- ○ Grounded
- ○ Energized
- ○ Constricted
- ○ Agitated
- ○ Other:

WHAT DO I WANT TO CONTINUE NOTICING OR DOING?

WHAT INSIGHTS AND OBSERVATIONS DO I WANT TO COME BACK TO?

WEEK SIX

WHERE I BELONG

The COVID-19 pandemic gave us an opportunity to reconsider our social networks and to identify which connections and friendships are the most rewarding and fulfilling for us.

Taking an intentional break from community during her microdosing journey allowed Shin Yu to examine her connections and determine which ones drained her and which ones brought her joy. Alliances once born out of survival—like high school friendships or pacts formed with colleagues from old jobs, relationships sometimes forged through gossip and negativity—receded into the past. She trimmed her social circles and disengaged from people who liked to provoke arguments or demand attention in her social media feeds.

As the pandemic wore on, Shin Yu's peers embraced ambitions to finish novels, renovate or redecorate their houses, or use their time "productively." Meanwhile, her son's year and a half of remote learning required her full attention. Catch-up conversations with friends often highlighted the differences between the daily lives of people who have children and those who don't. These interactions made her feel anxious, stuck, and unproductive. As the world contracted, she had to find a way to be at ease within her own immediate circumstances, to embrace deeply the specificity of her own life.

So she joined an online meditation group, where she found a deeper sense of just being, without doing or wanting. Through this practice, it became easier to be with thoughts about herself and about others without judgment. Comparing ourselves with others is exhausting and an obstacle to authentic connection.

Sometimes you have to turn the gaze inward to see more clearly the spaces where you feel a sense of welcome. That sense of acceptance might come from being with yourself, in a meditation group, or in a different social group, depending on where your intuition guides you.

How can your microdosing assist you in growing your self-awareness and your situational awareness and making choices that support a sense of belonging?

INQUIRIES

What do you lose or gain by making yourself conform to the expectations of others?

How do your social connections honor and respect your true self and spirit? How do you honor and respect the true self and spirit of your friends and family?

In what situations have you avoided sharing your full self? When have you hidden parts of yourself?

What does it feel like to take off the mask?

INSIGHTS AND OBSERVATIONS

DATE:

MY OVERALL MOOD IS:

- ○ Neutral
- ○ Curious
- ○ Irritated
- ○ Calm
- ○ Worried
- ○ Excited
- ○ Burnt Out
- ○ Preoccupied
- ○ Contemplative
- ○ Other:

THE EMOTIONS I FEEL TODAY ARE:

- ○ Happiness
- ○ Frustration
- ○ Sadness
- ○ Anger
- ○ Peace
- ○ Apathy
- ○ Overwhelm
- ○ Other:

MY BODY FEELS:

- ○ Heavy
- ○ Light
- ○ Relaxed
- ○ Alert
- ○ Grounded
- ○ Energized
- ○ Constricted
- ○ Agitated
- ○ Other:

WHAT DO I WANT TO CONTINUE NOTICING OR DOING?

WHAT INSIGHTS AND OBSERVATIONS DO I WANT TO COME BACK TO?

INSIGHTS AND OBSERVATIONS

DATE:

MY OVERALL MOOD IS:

- ◯ Neutral
- ◯ Curious
- ◯ Irritated
- ◯ Calm
- ◯ Worried
- ◯ Excited
- ◯ Burnt Out
- ◯ Preoccupied
- ◯ Contemplative
- ◯ Other:

THE EMOTIONS I FEEL TODAY ARE:

- ◯ Happiness
- ◯ Frustration
- ◯ Sadness
- ◯ Anger
- ◯ Peace
- ◯ Apathy
- ◯ Overwhelm
- ◯ Other:

MY BODY FEELS:

- ◯ Heavy
- ◯ Light
- ◯ Relaxed
- ◯ Alert
- ◯ Grounded
- ◯ Energized
- ◯ Constricted
- ◯ Agitated
- ◯ Other:

WHAT DO I WANT TO CONTINUE NOTICING OR DOING?

WHAT INSIGHTS AND OBSERVATIONS DO I WANT TO COME BACK TO?

INSIGHTS AND OBSERVATIONS

DATE:

MY OVERALL MOOD IS:
- ○ Neutral
- ○ Curious
- ○ Irritated
- ○ Calm
- ○ Worried
- ○ Excited
- ○ Burnt Out
- ○ Preoccupied
- ○ Contemplative
- ○ Other: _____

THE EMOTIONS I FEEL TODAY ARE:
- ○ Happiness
- ○ Frustration
- ○ Sadness
- ○ Anger
- ○ Peace
- ○ Apathy
- ○ Overwhelm
- ○ Other: _____

MY BODY FEELS:
- ○ Heavy
- ○ Light
- ○ Relaxed
- ○ Alert
- ○ Grounded
- ○ Energized
- ○ Constricted
- ○ Agitated
- ○ Other: _____

WHAT DO I WANT TO CONTINUE NOTICING OR DOING?

WHAT INSIGHTS AND OBSERVATIONS DO I WANT TO COME BACK TO?

INSIGHTS AND OBSERVATIONS

DATE:

MY OVERALL MOOD IS:

- ○ Neutral
- ○ Curious
- ○ Irritated
- ○ Calm
- ○ Worried
- ○ Excited
- ○ Burnt Out
- ○ Preoccupied
- ○ Contemplative
- ○ Other:

THE EMOTIONS I FEEL TODAY ARE:

- ○ Happiness
- ○ Frustration
- ○ Sadness
- ○ Anger
- ○ Peace
- ○ Apathy
- ○ Overwhelm
- ○ Other:

MY BODY FEELS:

- ○ Heavy
- ○ Light
- ○ Relaxed
- ○ Alert
- ○ Grounded
- ○ Energized
- ○ Constricted
- ○ Agitated
- ○ Other:

WHAT DO I WANT TO CONTINUE NOTICING OR DOING?

WHAT INSIGHTS AND OBSERVATIONS DO I WANT TO COME BACK TO?

INSIGHTS AND OBSERVATIONS

DATE:

MY OVERALL MOOD IS:

- ○ Neutral
- ○ Curious
- ○ Irritated
- ○ Calm
- ○ Worried
- ○ Excited
- ○ Burnt Out
- ○ Preoccupied
- ○ Contemplative
- ○ Other:

THE EMOTIONS I FEEL TODAY ARE:

- ○ Happiness
- ○ Frustration
- ○ Sadness
- ○ Anger
- ○ Peace
- ○ Apathy
- ○ Overwhelm
- ○ Other:

MY BODY FEELS:

- ○ Heavy
- ○ Light
- ○ Relaxed
- ○ Alert
- ○ Grounded
- ○ Energized
- ○ Constricted
- ○ Agitated
- ○ Other:

WHAT DO I WANT TO CONTINUE NOTICING OR DOING?

WHAT INSIGHTS AND OBSERVATIONS DO I WANT TO COME BACK TO?

WEEK SEVEN

THE ART OF
NOT DOING

Throughout Amy's childhood and young adulthood, anxiety ruled her thoughts and behaviors. When there was a problem, she rushed to fix it. This was doubly true when a rift occurred in any of her relationships. Her default reaction in these situations was to be an apologizing people pleaser.

Microdosing with psychedelics allowed her to recognize that this anxiety was her way of protecting herself from slowing down enough to feel shame or the judgment of others. These days, microdosing is one of many awareness tools she uses to analyze what she's doing to support her authentic self.

Many years ago, Amy and her brother became estranged. In Chinese families that prioritize clan harmony, estrangement is particularly serious. Her anxiety about the rift with her brother became an alarm clock that woke her every night to work on the problem. But when we're in emotional distress, we're at our least effective at solving problems and thinking coherently.

Her meditation teacher taught her to use a Hindu mantra. Month by month, it helped her shift her attachment away from anxious thoughts. Instead, she focused on the Sanskrit syllables and sounds of the mantra. She pondered the meaning of the mantra and the fact that it had been passed down through the centuries to this moment in time. She practiced aloud in her meditation space and silently everywhere else. One night, when her anxiety woke her again, the mantra surprised her. It was the first thought to fill her mind, rather than the rumination. In that moment, pivoting to the mantra helped her loosen the grip of anxiety, her default mode network. Doing the mantra practice helped her "not do" the anxiety.

Integrating insights from microdosing and other experiences is one of the many practices Amy does each day, from moment to moment, to help her not do something out of anxiety, so that she can do what is vital and supports her living life authentically.

What practices help you with "not doing" or disengaging from your default ways of being?

INQUIRIES

What do you feel compelled or obligated
to do that you can stop doing?

What gives you permission to not
do that thing?

How difficult or easy is it to not engage
with this behavior?

What arises out of the process of not doing?

What happens when you stop multitasking and
instead focus on doing one thing at a time?

INSIGHTS AND OBSERVATIONS

DATE:

MY OVERALL MOOD IS:
- ○ Neutral
- ○ Curious
- ○ Irritated
- ○ Calm
- ○ Worried
- ○ Excited
- ○ Burnt Out
- ○ Preoccupied
- ○ Contemplative
- ○ Other: _____

THE EMOTIONS I FEEL TODAY ARE:
- ○ Happiness
- ○ Frustration
- ○ Sadness
- ○ Anger
- ○ Peace
- ○ Apathy
- ○ Overwhelm
- ○ Other: _____

MY BODY FEELS:
- ○ Heavy
- ○ Light
- ○ Relaxed
- ○ Alert
- ○ Grounded
- ○ Energized
- ○ Constricted
- ○ Agitated
- ○ Other: _____

WHAT DO I WANT TO CONTINUE NOTICING OR DOING?

WHAT INSIGHTS AND OBSERVATIONS DO I WANT TO COME BACK TO?

INSIGHTS AND OBSERVATIONS

DATE:

MY OVERALL MOOD IS:
- Neutral
- Curious
- Irritated
- Calm
- Worried
- Excited
- Burnt Out
- Preoccupied
- Contemplative
- Other:

THE EMOTIONS I FEEL TODAY ARE:
- Happiness
- Frustration
- Sadness
- Anger
- Peace
- Apathy
- Overwhelm
- Other:

MY BODY FEELS:
- Heavy
- Light
- Relaxed
- Alert
- Grounded
- Energized
- Constricted
- Agitated
- Other:

WHAT DO I WANT TO CONTINUE NOTICING OR DOING?

WHAT INSIGHTS AND OBSERVATIONS DO I WANT TO COME BACK TO?

INSIGHTS AND OBSERVATIONS

DATE:

MY OVERALL MOOD IS:

- ○ Neutral
- ○ Curious
- ○ Irritated
- ○ Calm
- ○ Worried
- ○ Excited
- ○ Burnt Out
- ○ Preoccupied
- ○ Contemplative
- ○ Other:

THE EMOTIONS I FEEL TODAY ARE:

- ○ Happiness
- ○ Frustration
- ○ Sadness
- ○ Anger
- ○ Peace
- ○ Apathy
- ○ Overwhelm
- ○ Other:

MY BODY FEELS:

- ○ Heavy
- ○ Light
- ○ Relaxed
- ○ Alert
- ○ Grounded
- ○ Energized
- ○ Constricted
- ○ Agitated
- ○ Other:

WHAT DO I WANT TO CONTINUE NOTICING OR DOING?

WHAT INSIGHTS AND OBSERVATIONS DO I WANT TO COME BACK TO?

INSIGHTS AND OBSERVATIONS

DATE:

MY OVERALL MOOD IS:
- ○ Neutral
- ○ Curious
- ○ Irritated
- ○ Calm
- ○ Worried
- ○ Excited
- ○ Burnt Out
- ○ Preoccupied
- ○ Contemplative
- ○ Other:

THE EMOTIONS I FEEL TODAY ARE:
- ○ Happiness
- ○ Frustration
- ○ Sadness
- ○ Anger
- ○ Peace
- ○ Apathy
- ○ Overwhelm
- ○ Other:

MY BODY FEELS:
- ○ Heavy
- ○ Light
- ○ Relaxed
- ○ Alert
- ○ Grounded
- ○ Energized
- ○ Constricted
- ○ Agitated
- ○ Other:

WHAT DO I WANT TO CONTINUE NOTICING OR DOING?

WHAT INSIGHTS AND OBSERVATIONS DO I WANT TO COME BACK TO?

INSIGHTS AND OBSERVATIONS

DATE:

MY OVERALL MOOD IS:

- ◯ Neutral
- ◯ Curious
- ◯ Irritated
- ◯ Calm
- ◯ Worried
- ◯ Excited
- ◯ Burnt Out
- ◯ Preoccupied
- ◯ Contemplative
- ◯ Other:

THE EMOTIONS I FEEL TODAY ARE:

- ◯ Happiness
- ◯ Frustration
- ◯ Sadness
- ◯ Anger
- ◯ Peace
- ◯ Apathy
- ◯ Overwhelm
- ◯ Other:

MY BODY FEELS:

- ◯ Heavy
- ◯ Light
- ◯ Relaxed
- ◯ Alert
- ◯ Grounded
- ◯ Energized
- ◯ Constricted
- ◯ Agitated
- ◯ Other:

WHAT DO I WANT TO CONTINUE NOTICING OR DOING?

WHAT INSIGHTS AND OBSERVATIONS DO I WANT TO COME BACK TO?

WEEK EIGHT

THE ART OF DOING

Last week, you worked to name and put aside behaviors and activities that don't serve you. Now you'll identify personal habits and behaviors that build stronger connections with your whole self.

Through the experience of microdosing, you've had a chance to explore isolating and leaning into your individual senses (Week Two). Take what you learned from those exercises and apply that same attention to everyday activities and actions. What do you notice when you're fully engaged in eating slowly and mindfully or taking a walk without a destination? What does it feel like to drink a hot beverage without burning your tongue? Or to wash dishes under warm water? Or to sink your hands into laundry pulled right out of the dryer? Make a list of everyday actions that bring pleasure.

Spend some time, too, getting in touch with discomfort. When a person first learns to meditate, they will likely be instructed to refrain from scratching an itch or moving a foot or leg that's gone numb. We notice and observe our discomfort to allow the mind to move past it. Discomfort can be a great teacher, as it's *not* the same as pain. It often exists to give us valuable information about where inner and outer experiences don't align. Fatigue and exhaustion are also important states to observe and know more about.

We've compiled a short list of activities and behaviors that we've found interesting to dive into from microdose to microdose. These include taking a voice lesson and paying attention to the vibration of the vocal cords during singing; noticing the sensation when a self-protective instinct kicks in and really paying attention to those physiological responses in the body; and shifting the mind toward focusing on what brings us pleasure or gratitude—centering our own experience and minding our own business—instead of projecting judgmental narratives onto others.

Whatever you put on the list of things that you want to do more of, know that your opportunities for insight aren't limited to your choice of activity. When you enter into being present with whatever you're doing, you carry with you a mindset of curiosity.

What has microdosing revealed to you about disrupting your usual routines? What practices, habits, or experiences can help you explore and nourish neglected parts of your own identity? Where can you bring curiosity into your daily life?

INQUIRIES

What are some things you can do to self-soothe when you're feeling overwhelmed or overstimulated?

What are you choosing to do in the space that you made by "not doing" last week?

How do you engage in intentional behaviors, thoughts, and emotions?

Where can you bring gratitude into the course of your daily life?

INSIGHTS AND OBSERVATIONS

DATE:

MY OVERALL MOOD IS:
- ○ Neutral
- ○ Curious
- ○ Irritated
- ○ Calm
- ○ Worried
- ○ Excited
- ○ Burnt Out
- ○ Preoccupied
- ○ Contemplative
- ○ Other:

THE EMOTIONS I FEEL TODAY ARE:
- ○ Happiness
- ○ Frustration
- ○ Sadness
- ○ Anger
- ○ Peace
- ○ Apathy
- ○ Overwhelm
- ○ Other:

MY BODY FEELS:
- ○ Heavy
- ○ Light
- ○ Relaxed
- ○ Alert
- ○ Grounded
- ○ Energized
- ○ Constricted
- ○ Agitated
- ○ Other:

WHAT DO I WANT TO CONTINUE NOTICING OR DOING?

WHAT INSIGHTS AND OBSERVATIONS DO I WANT TO COME BACK TO?

INSIGHTS AND OBSERVATIONS

DATE:

MY OVERALL MOOD IS:

- ○ Neutral
- ○ Curious
- ○ Irritated
- ○ Calm
- ○ Worried
- ○ Excited
- ○ Burnt Out
- ○ Preoccupied
- ○ Contemplative
- ○ Other:

THE EMOTIONS I FEEL TODAY ARE:

- ○ Happiness
- ○ Frustration
- ○ Sadness
- ○ Anger
- ○ Peace
- ○ Apathy
- ○ Overwhelm
- ○ Other:

MY BODY FEELS:

- ○ Heavy
- ○ Light
- ○ Relaxed
- ○ Alert
- ○ Grounded
- ○ Energized
- ○ Constricted
- ○ Agitated
- ○ Other:

WHAT DO I WANT TO CONTINUE NOTICING OR DOING?

WHAT INSIGHTS AND OBSERVATIONS DO I WANT TO COME BACK TO?

INSIGHTS AND OBSERVATIONS

DATE:

MY OVERALL MOOD IS:

- ○ Neutral
- ○ Curious
- ○ Irritated
- ○ Calm
- ○ Worried
- ○ Excited
- ○ Burnt Out
- ○ Preoccupied
- ○ Contemplative
- ○ Other:

THE EMOTIONS I FEEL TODAY ARE:

- ○ Happiness
- ○ Frustration
- ○ Sadness
- ○ Anger
- ○ Peace
- ○ Apathy
- ○ Overwhelm
- ○ Other:

MY BODY FEELS:

- ○ Heavy
- ○ Light
- ○ Relaxed
- ○ Alert
- ○ Grounded
- ○ Energized
- ○ Constricted
- ○ Agitated
- ○ Other:

WHAT DO I WANT TO CONTINUE NOTICING OR DOING?

WHAT INSIGHTS AND OBSERVATIONS DO I WANT TO COME BACK TO?

INSIGHTS AND OBSERVATIONS

DATE:

MY OVERALL MOOD IS:

- ○ Neutral
- ○ Curious
- ○ Irritated
- ○ Calm
- ○ Worried
- ○ Excited
- ○ Burnt Out
- ○ Preoccupied
- ○ Contemplative
- ○ Other:

THE EMOTIONS I FEEL TODAY ARE:

- ○ Happiness
- ○ Frustration
- ○ Sadness
- ○ Anger
- ○ Peace
- ○ Apathy
- ○ Overwhelm
- ○ Other:

MY BODY FEELS:

- ○ Heavy
- ○ Light
- ○ Relaxed
- ○ Alert
- ○ Grounded
- ○ Energized
- ○ Constricted
- ○ Agitated
- ○ Other:

WHAT DO I WANT TO CONTINUE NOTICING OR DOING?

WHAT INSIGHTS AND OBSERVATIONS DO I WANT TO COME BACK TO?

INSIGHTS AND OBSERVATIONS

DATE:

MY OVERALL MOOD IS:

- ◯ Neutral
- ◯ Curious
- ◯ Irritated
- ◯ Calm
- ◯ Worried
- ◯ Excited
- ◯ Burnt Out
- ◯ Preoccupied
- ◯ Contemplative
- ◯ Other:

THE EMOTIONS I FEEL TODAY ARE:

- ◯ Happiness
- ◯ Frustration
- ◯ Sadness
- ◯ Anger
- ◯ Peace
- ◯ Apathy
- ◯ Overwhelm
- ◯ Other:

MY BODY FEELS:

- ◯ Heavy
- ◯ Light
- ◯ Relaxed
- ◯ Alert
- ◯ Grounded
- ◯ Energized
- ◯ Constricted
- ◯ Agitated
- ◯ Other:

WHAT DO I WANT TO CONTINUE NOTICING OR DOING?

WHAT INSIGHTS AND OBSERVATIONS DO I WANT TO COME BACK TO?

WEEK NINE

MY FOUNDATION AND WHO SHAPED IT

Modern life requires that we continually update and innovate our lifestyles to suit the times in which we're living. Our present-day experiences can include cloud-based virtual assistants, grocery stores with no cashiers, QR code menus, and other automated systems that take us further and further away from personal connection. Our bonds to community and public spaces erode, and our human-to-human connection fades.

It's easy to lose the connection to older traditions and other ways of being. Across generations, labor opportunities, war, famine, and exile have created some of the conditions for migration and immigration. When these life-altering shifts take place, markers of identity—including family and social structures, language, land, and community—can be lost. To survive, a person may feel compelled to choose between assimilation into a new culture and holding on to the core parts of their original identity.

How can we honor cultural bereavement and recover a connection to our ancestors, their traditions, and knowledge? How can understanding our family origins and history give us insight and gratitude for who we are in this present life? How can our inquiry encourage intergenerational healing and honor and celebrate the legacies of those who came before us?

INQUIRIES

What are the cultural and familial practices and traditions that form your foundation?

How is your life similar to or different from the lives of your ancestors?

What are some of the ways in which you'd like to stay connected to your ancestors?

What are some of the ways in which you'd like to continue learning more about your ancestors?

How do your ancestors or ancestral traditions support your authentic identity now?

How do you wish to imprint your legacy in the world through your actions and responses?

INSIGHTS AND OBSERVATIONS

DATE:

MY OVERALL MOOD IS:
- ○ Neutral
- ○ Curious
- ○ Irritated
- ○ Calm
- ○ Worried
- ○ Excited
- ○ Burnt Out
- ○ Preoccupied
- ○ Contemplative
- ○ Other:

THE EMOTIONS I FEEL TODAY ARE:
- ○ Happiness
- ○ Frustration
- ○ Sadness
- ○ Anger
- ○ Peace
- ○ Apathy
- ○ Overwhelm
- ○ Other:

MY BODY FEELS:
- ○ Heavy
- ○ Light
- ○ Relaxed
- ○ Alert
- ○ Grounded
- ○ Energized
- ○ Constricted
- ○ Agitated
- ○ Other:

WHAT DO I WANT TO CONTINUE NOTICING OR DOING?

WHAT INSIGHTS AND OBSERVATIONS DO I WANT TO COME BACK TO?

INSIGHTS AND OBSERVATIONS

DATE:

MY OVERALL MOOD IS:
- ◯ Neutral
- ◯ Curious
- ◯ Irritated
- ◯ Calm
- ◯ Worried
- ◯ Excited
- ◯ Burnt Out
- ◯ Preoccupied
- ◯ Contemplative
- ◯ Other:

THE EMOTIONS I FEEL TODAY ARE:
- ◯ Happiness
- ◯ Frustration
- ◯ Sadness
- ◯ Anger
- ◯ Peace
- ◯ Apathy
- ◯ Overwhelm
- ◯ Other:

MY BODY FEELS:
- ◯ Heavy
- ◯ Light
- ◯ Relaxed
- ◯ Alert
- ◯ Grounded
- ◯ Energized
- ◯ Constricted
- ◯ Agitated
- ◯ Other:

WHAT DO I WANT TO CONTINUE NOTICING OR DOING?

WHAT INSIGHTS AND OBSERVATIONS DO I WANT TO COME BACK TO?

INSIGHTS AND OBSERVATIONS

DATE:

MY OVERALL MOOD IS:
- ○ Neutral
- ○ Curious
- ○ Irritated
- ○ Calm
- ○ Worried
- ○ Excited
- ○ Burnt Out
- ○ Preoccupied
- ○ Contemplative
- ○ Other:

THE EMOTIONS I FEEL TODAY ARE:
- ○ Happiness
- ○ Frustration
- ○ Sadness
- ○ Anger
- ○ Peace
- ○ Apathy
- ○ Overwhelm
- ○ Other:

MY BODY FEELS:
- ○ Heavy
- ○ Light
- ○ Relaxed
- ○ Alert
- ○ Grounded
- ○ Energized
- ○ Constricted
- ○ Agitated
- ○ Other:

WHAT DO I WANT TO CONTINUE NOTICING OR DOING?

WHAT INSIGHTS AND OBSERVATIONS DO I WANT TO COME BACK TO?

INSIGHTS AND OBSERVATIONS

DATE:

MY OVERALL MOOD IS:
- ○ Neutral
- ○ Curious
- ○ Irritated
- ○ Calm
- ○ Worried
- ○ Excited
- ○ Burnt Out
- ○ Preoccupied
- ○ Contemplative
- ○ Other:

THE EMOTIONS I FEEL TODAY ARE:
- ○ Happiness
- ○ Frustration
- ○ Sadness
- ○ Anger
- ○ Peace
- ○ Apathy
- ○ Overwhelm
- ○ Other:

MY BODY FEELS:
- ○ Heavy
- ○ Light
- ○ Relaxed
- ○ Alert
- ○ Grounded
- ○ Energized
- ○ Constricted
- ○ Agitated
- ○ Other:

WHAT DO I WANT TO CONTINUE NOTICING OR DOING?

WHAT INSIGHTS AND OBSERVATIONS DO I WANT TO COME BACK TO?

INSIGHTS AND OBSERVATIONS

DATE:

MY OVERALL MOOD IS:
- ○ Neutral
- ○ Curious
- ○ Irritated
- ○ Calm
- ○ Worried
- ○ Excited
- ○ Burnt Out
- ○ Preoccupied
- ○ Contemplative
- ○ Other: _____

THE EMOTIONS I FEEL TODAY ARE:
- ○ Happiness
- ○ Frustration
- ○ Sadness
- ○ Anger
- ○ Peace
- ○ Apathy
- ○ Overwhelm
- ○ Other: _____

MY BODY FEELS:
- ○ Heavy
- ○ Light
- ○ Relaxed
- ○ Alert
- ○ Grounded
- ○ Energized
- ○ Constricted
- ○ Agitated
- ○ Other: _____

WHAT DO I WANT TO CONTINUE NOTICING OR DOING?

WHAT INSIGHTS AND OBSERVATIONS DO I WANT TO COME BACK TO?

WEEK TEN

WHAT I WANT TO ANCHOR IN

As you reflect on your journey with microdosing, tap into your curiosity to process your observations. Think about what stands out in your experiences. This week, like the remaining sections of this journal, invites you to consolidate your knowledge.

Theories on psychological development all have one thing in common: They all define periods of challenge, followed by periods of perspective on lessons learned. People who were not supported in healthy ways during one or more of their developmental stages experience those challenges in subsequent stages and in their adult identity. This is why psychotherapy is a long-term undertaking. Care must be taken to consider how those challenges are addressed.

During your microdosing journey, what challenged what you thought you knew about yourself, your relationships, your purpose, and your identity? What became essential for you to do or no longer do? What did you learn about who you prioritized in relationships and other experiences?

Earlier, we invited you into the challenge of noticing where alignment and misalignment exist for you. You explored habits and behaviors that you adopted or assumed. Now we invite you to write down what you have learned about yourself.

For Amy, turning fifty has offered a chance to reflect on her past decades of experience. In the midpoint of her life, the microdosing experience has revealed the small doses of knowledge that show up every day, if she slows down enough to pay attention. Microdosing has helped her develop practices, rituals, and routines to slow her mind down and to keep it healthy. Many of these have become moment-to-moment practices. Modern daily life is not easy, but Amy wants to approach life with grace, flow, pleasure, and joy—to make room for creativity and to deliberately commit time and effort to liberating herself from conditioning that impedes these experiences.

As you work through what you want to consolidate from your microdosing journey, survey your experiences over the past few months. What questions or intentions led you to the microdosing journey in the first place? What changed for you during this journey, and what did you learn? What seeds from this experience do you wish to plant in your soil?

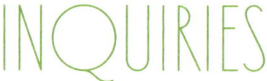

What are some of the intentions and goals that you set during your microdosing journey?

What is one new thing that you learned about yourself or how you think? How does this self-discovery change how you see yourself or the world?

How else have you changed over the past ten weeks? What new insights, behaviors, and responses stand out to you?

Where are you curious, energized, or hopeful?

Is there anything that you're ready to let go of? If so, what and why?

INSIGHTS AND OBSERVATIONS

DATE:

MY OVERALL MOOD IS:

- ○ Neutral
- ○ Curious
- ○ Irritated
- ○ Calm
- ○ Worried
- ○ Excited
- ○ Burnt Out
- ○ Preoccupied
- ○ Contemplative
- ○ Other:

THE EMOTIONS I FEEL TODAY ARE:

- ○ Happiness
- ○ Frustration
- ○ Sadness
- ○ Anger
- ○ Peace
- ○ Apathy
- ○ Overwhelm
- ○ Other:

MY BODY FEELS:

- ○ Heavy
- ○ Light
- ○ Relaxed
- ○ Alert
- ○ Grounded
- ○ Energized
- ○ Constricted
- ○ Agitated
- ○ Other:

WHAT DO I WANT TO CONTINUE NOTICING OR DOING?

WHAT INSIGHTS AND OBSERVATIONS DO I WANT TO COME BACK TO?

INSIGHTS AND OBSERVATIONS

DATE:

MY OVERALL MOOD IS:
- ○ Neutral
- ○ Curious
- ○ Irritated
- ○ Calm
- ○ Worried
- ○ Excited
- ○ Burnt Out
- ○ Preoccupied
- ○ Contemplative
- ○ Other:

THE EMOTIONS I FEEL TODAY ARE:
- ○ Happiness
- ○ Frustration
- ○ Sadness
- ○ Anger
- ○ Peace
- ○ Apathy
- ○ Overwhelm
- ○ Other:

MY BODY FEELS:
- ○ Heavy
- ○ Light
- ○ Relaxed
- ○ Alert
- ○ Grounded
- ○ Energized
- ○ Constricted
- ○ Agitated
- ○ Other:

WHAT DO I WANT TO CONTINUE NOTICING OR DOING?

WHAT INSIGHTS AND OBSERVATIONS DO I WANT TO COME BACK TO?

INSIGHTS AND OBSERVATIONS

DATE:

MY OVERALL MOOD IS:
- ◯ Neutral
- ◯ Curious
- ◯ Irritated
- ◯ Calm
- ◯ Worried
- ◯ Excited
- ◯ Burnt Out
- ◯ Preoccupied
- ◯ Contemplative
- ◯ Other:

THE EMOTIONS I FEEL TODAY ARE:
- ◯ Happiness
- ◯ Frustration
- ◯ Sadness
- ◯ Anger
- ◯ Peace
- ◯ Apathy
- ◯ Overwhelm
- ◯ Other:

MY BODY FEELS:
- ◯ Heavy
- ◯ Light
- ◯ Relaxed
- ◯ Alert
- ◯ Grounded
- ◯ Energized
- ◯ Constricted
- ◯ Agitated
- ◯ Other:

WHAT DO I WANT TO CONTINUE NOTICING OR DOING?

WHAT INSIGHTS AND OBSERVATIONS DO I WANT TO COME BACK TO?

INSIGHTS AND OBSERVATIONS

DATE:

MY OVERALL MOOD IS:
- ○ Neutral
- ○ Curious
- ○ Irritated
- ○ Calm
- ○ Worried
- ○ Excited
- ○ Burnt Out
- ○ Preoccupied
- ○ Contemplative
- ○ Other:

THE EMOTIONS I FEEL TODAY ARE:
- ○ Happiness
- ○ Frustration
- ○ Sadness
- ○ Anger
- ○ Peace
- ○ Apathy
- ○ Overwhelm
- ○ Other:

MY BODY FEELS:
- ○ Heavy
- ○ Light
- ○ Relaxed
- ○ Alert
- ○ Grounded
- ○ Energized
- ○ Constricted
- ○ Agitated
- ○ Other:

WHAT DO I WANT TO CONTINUE NOTICING OR DOING?

WHAT INSIGHTS AND OBSERVATIONS DO I WANT TO COME BACK TO?

INSIGHTS AND OBSERVATIONS

DATE:

MY OVERALL MOOD IS:

- ○ Neutral
- ○ Curious
- ○ Irritated
- ○ Calm
- ○ Worried
- ○ Excited
- ○ Burnt Out
- ○ Preoccupied
- ○ Contemplative
- ○ Other:

THE EMOTIONS I FEEL TODAY ARE:

- ○ Happiness
- ○ Frustration
- ○ Sadness
- ○ Anger
- ○ Peace
- ○ Apathy
- ○ Overwhelm
- ○ Other:

MY BODY FEELS:

- ○ Heavy
- ○ Light
- ○ Relaxed
- ○ Alert
- ○ Grounded
- ○ Energized
- ○ Constricted
- ○ Agitated
- ○ Other:

WHAT DO I WANT TO CONTINUE NOTICING OR DOING?

WHAT INSIGHTS AND OBSERVATIONS DO I WANT TO COME BACK TO?

WEEK ELEVEN

HOLDING THE SELF IN THE WORLD DIFFERENTLY

When Shin Yu first began microdosing, she kept a daily journal that documented all her dosing and integration days. She wrote down emotional insights and deeply contemplated family and work conflicts with more curiosity. With her default mode network turned down, she could bring a less judgmental perspective to reimagining old narratives. She also recorded her physical and emotional reactions to various experiences and became more intentional about managing her stress better.

Shin Yu continued this writing practice for nine months and then, as her work and personal schedules got busier, she stopped. She didn't stop microdosing, but after writing down her microdosing experiences for most of the year, she found herself practicing and integrating new habits without needing to track them.

When we embark on a meditation practice, we explore a form that supports us in being consistent and intentional. By putting aside protected time and space, we create a setting in which we can begin to practice being more present. But it's misleading to think that the practice of presence *only* happens on the meditation cushion or that it occurs separately from our everyday lives. Ask a Zen teacher how many hours they meditate a day, and they might answer, "None." Or they might tell you, "I'm meditating right now." Both are true.

There is more than one path to mindfulness. Microdosing, journaling, and meditation are just a few forms that help us come into better awareness. But we can take our practice beyond the microdose, meditation studio, or page and into our everyday lives. The ultimate goal is to let go of form so that inner peace becomes possible in any state. By becoming embodied in our experience, we realize that we are not separate from the world. And when we know this truth, we hold ourselves differently.

INQUIRIES

List the practices that you explored during your microdosing journey that you'd like to keep doing.

Make a list of beliefs or behaviors that you're ready to retire.

What changes do you need in your life, work, or relationships right now? What do those changes look like in the short term? And in the long term?

How has better awareness of your behaviors and tendencies in the world helped you make different choices?

What strengths have revealed themselves as you overcame challenges? Where have you developed resiliency?

What permissions do you need to give yourself to say yes? To say no?

INSIGHTS AND OBSERVATIONS

DATE:

MY OVERALL MOOD IS:
- ○ Neutral
- ○ Curious
- ○ Irritated
- ○ Calm
- ○ Worried
- ○ Excited
- ○ Burnt Out
- ○ Preoccupied
- ○ Contemplative
- ○ Other:

THE EMOTIONS I FEEL TODAY ARE:
- ○ Happiness
- ○ Frustration
- ○ Sadness
- ○ Anger
- ○ Peace
- ○ Apathy
- ○ Overwhelm
- ○ Other:

MY BODY FEELS:
- ○ Heavy
- ○ Light
- ○ Relaxed
- ○ Alert
- ○ Grounded
- ○ Energized
- ○ Constricted
- ○ Agitated
- ○ Other:

WHAT DO I WANT TO CONTINUE NOTICING OR DOING?

WHAT INSIGHTS AND OBSERVATIONS DO I WANT TO COME BACK TO?

INSIGHTS AND OBSERVATIONS

DATE:

MY OVERALL MOOD IS:

- ◯ Neutral
- ◯ Curious
- ◯ Irritated
- ◯ Calm
- ◯ Worried
- ◯ Excited
- ◯ Burnt Out
- ◯ Preoccupied
- ◯ Contemplative
- ◯ Other: _____

THE EMOTIONS I FEEL TODAY ARE:

- ◯ Happiness
- ◯ Frustration
- ◯ Sadness
- ◯ Anger
- ◯ Peace
- ◯ Apathy
- ◯ Overwhelm
- ◯ Other: _____

MY BODY FEELS:

- ◯ Heavy
- ◯ Light
- ◯ Relaxed
- ◯ Alert
- ◯ Grounded
- ◯ Energized
- ◯ Constricted
- ◯ Agitated
- ◯ Other: _____

WHAT DO I WANT TO CONTINUE NOTICING OR DOING?

WHAT INSIGHTS AND OBSERVATIONS DO I WANT TO COME BACK TO?

INSIGHTS AND OBSERVATIONS

DATE:

MY OVERALL MOOD IS:

- ◯ Neutral
- ◯ Curious
- ◯ Irritated
- ◯ Calm
- ◯ Worried
- ◯ Excited
- ◯ Burnt Out
- ◯ Preoccupied
- ◯ Contemplative
- ◯ Other: _____

THE EMOTIONS I FEEL TODAY ARE:

- ◯ Happiness
- ◯ Frustration
- ◯ Sadness
- ◯ Anger
- ◯ Peace
- ◯ Apathy
- ◯ Overwhelm
- ◯ Other: _____

MY BODY FEELS:

- ◯ Heavy
- ◯ Light
- ◯ Relaxed
- ◯ Alert
- ◯ Grounded
- ◯ Energized
- ◯ Constricted
- ◯ Agitated
- ◯ Other: _____

WHAT DO I WANT TO CONTINUE NOTICING OR DOING?

_____
_____
_____

WHAT INSIGHTS AND OBSERVATIONS DO I WANT TO COME BACK TO?

_____
_____
_____

INSIGHTS AND OBSERVATIONS

DATE:

MY OVERALL MOOD IS:
- ○ Neutral
- ○ Curious
- ○ Irritated
- ○ Calm
- ○ Worried
- ○ Excited
- ○ Burnt Out
- ○ Preoccupied
- ○ Contemplative
- ○ Other:

THE EMOTIONS I FEEL TODAY ARE:
- ○ Happiness
- ○ Frustration
- ○ Sadness
- ○ Anger
- ○ Peace
- ○ Apathy
- ○ Overwhelm
- ○ Other:

MY BODY FEELS:
- ○ Heavy
- ○ Light
- ○ Relaxed
- ○ Alert
- ○ Grounded
- ○ Energized
- ○ Constricted
- ○ Agitated
- ○ Other:

WHAT DO I WANT TO CONTINUE NOTICING OR DOING?

WHAT INSIGHTS AND OBSERVATIONS DO I WANT TO COME BACK TO?

INSIGHTS AND OBSERVATIONS

DATE:

MY OVERALL MOOD IS:
- ○ Neutral
- ○ Curious
- ○ Irritated
- ○ Calm
- ○ Worried
- ○ Excited
- ○ Burnt Out
- ○ Preoccupied
- ○ Contemplative
- ○ Other: _____

THE EMOTIONS I FEEL TODAY ARE:
- ○ Happiness
- ○ Frustration
- ○ Sadness
- ○ Anger
- ○ Peace
- ○ Apathy
- ○ Overwhelm
- ○ Other: _____

MY BODY FEELS:
- ○ Heavy
- ○ Light
- ○ Relaxed
- ○ Alert
- ○ Grounded
- ○ Energized
- ○ Constricted
- ○ Agitated
- ○ Other: _____

WHAT DO I WANT TO CONTINUE NOTICING OR DOING?

_____

_____

WHAT INSIGHTS AND OBSERVATIONS DO I WANT TO COME BACK TO?

_____

_____

WEEK TWELVE AND BEYOND

AFTER MICRODOSING

In *The Language of Butterflies*, author Wendy Williams writes that when a monarch caterpillar goes into its chrysalis, the form that emerges—the monarch butterfly—can vary vastly based on what the caterpillar experiences during its larval stage. Caterpillars that experience harsh conditions (less sunlight, cold) emerge as butterflies with stronger, larger wingspans for long migrations, whereas those that experience hospitable conditions (longer days, warmth, humidity) emerge with brighter colors to attract mates.

During your microdosing journey, what environmental conditions have you felt, tasted, and heard? How did these factors and your awareness of them affect you over these three months? As you emerge from your work with this microdosing companion, what essential parts have you transformed?

During transformation, we must trust the process of change. If we are mindful and act intentionally, we hope for closer alignment with our values. During this process, which is sometimes difficult, often nonlinear, maybe even lifelong, it's easy to get lost. There is never one quick and simple fix that produces change. That's why we encourage you to build a tool kit of companion practices that support you in holding and embodying your intention.

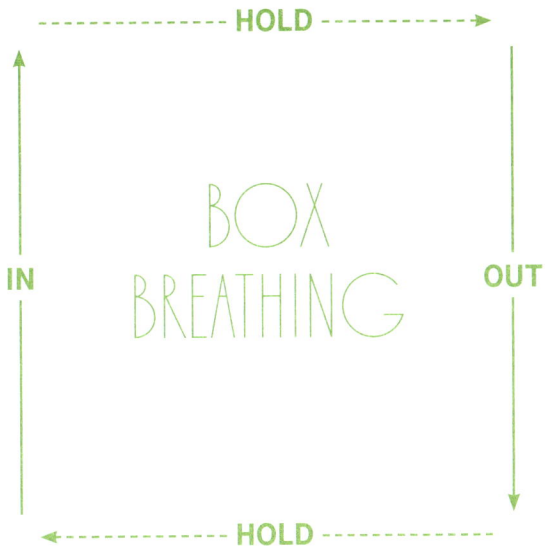

Navy SEALs use a technique called box breathing during tactical operations. One would think that in an intense, dangerous situation the last thing one could focus on is the breath. But it is essential. The body must be online in order for the mind to work. The Navy SEALs use their breath to resource their body with oxygen, but also because focused breath work balances the parasympathetic and sympathetic nervous systems. When the body is balanced, higher-order thinking such as cognition and emotion is more likely to be organized too.

Try box breathing for yourself. Inhale slowly for a count of four. Hold the breath for a count of four. Exhale slowly for a count of four. Now pause for a count of four. Repeat, starting with the inhale.

As humans, we often think with our minds and disregard our bodies' signals. But we can also make a conscious choice to pursue more balance. Here is an invitation to try this breathing exercise again. As you inhale, consider all that you have experienced these past three months. Hold it. Exhale slowly and consider all that you are letting go of and all the changes and shifts you have made. Pause and trust. What comes next?

How have you come to trust what you now know about yourself? How differently do you hear your inner voice, your authentic self? Where do you want to take action with your intentions?

INQUIRIES

What has changed for you about how you'd like to show up in the world?

How do you define self-care now versus at the beginning of your journey?

What intentions would you like to explore in the near and distant future?

What questions will continue to support you in loosening the grip of your default identities and roles?

What do you trust about yourself?

What do you feel is the most important takeaway from this experience?

INSIGHTS AND OBSERVATIONS

DATE:

MY OVERALL MOOD IS:
- ○ Neutral
- ○ Curious
- ○ Irritated
- ○ Calm
- ○ Worried
- ○ Excited
- ○ Burnt Out
- ○ Preoccupied
- ○ Contemplative
- ○ Other:

THE EMOTIONS I FEEL TODAY ARE:
- ○ Happiness
- ○ Frustration
- ○ Sadness
- ○ Anger
- ○ Peace
- ○ Apathy
- ○ Overwhelm
- ○ Other:

MY BODY FEELS:
- ○ Heavy
- ○ Light
- ○ Relaxed
- ○ Alert
- ○ Grounded
- ○ Energized
- ○ Constricted
- ○ Agitated
- ○ Other:

WHAT DO I WANT TO CONTINUE NOTICING OR DOING?

WHAT INSIGHTS AND OBSERVATIONS DO I WANT TO COME BACK TO?

INSIGHTS AND OBSERVATIONS

DATE:

MY OVERALL MOOD IS:

- ○ Neutral
- ○ Curious
- ○ Irritated
- ○ Calm
- ○ Worried
- ○ Excited
- ○ Burnt Out
- ○ Preoccupied
- ○ Contemplative
- ○ Other:

THE EMOTIONS I FEEL TODAY ARE:

- ○ Happiness
- ○ Frustration
- ○ Sadness
- ○ Anger
- ○ Peace
- ○ Apathy
- ○ Overwhelm
- ○ Other:

MY BODY FEELS:

- ○ Heavy
- ○ Light
- ○ Relaxed
- ○ Alert
- ○ Grounded
- ○ Energized
- ○ Constricted
- ○ Agitated
- ○ Other:

WHAT DO I WANT TO CONTINUE NOTICING OR DOING?

WHAT INSIGHTS AND OBSERVATIONS DO I WANT TO COME BACK TO?

INSIGHTS AND OBSERVATIONS

DATE:

MY OVERALL MOOD IS:

- ○ Neutral
- ○ Curious
- ○ Irritated
- ○ Calm
- ○ Worried
- ○ Excited
- ○ Burnt Out
- ○ Preoccupied
- ○ Contemplative
- ○ Other:

THE EMOTIONS I FEEL TODAY ARE:

- ○ Happiness
- ○ Frustration
- ○ Sadness
- ○ Anger
- ○ Peace
- ○ Apathy
- ○ Overwhelm
- ○ Other:

MY BODY FEELS:

- ○ Heavy
- ○ Light
- ○ Relaxed
- ○ Alert
- ○ Grounded
- ○ Energized
- ○ Constricted
- ○ Agitated
- ○ Other:

WHAT DO I WANT TO CONTINUE NOTICING OR DOING?

WHAT INSIGHTS AND OBSERVATIONS DO I WANT TO COME BACK TO?

INSIGHTS AND OBSERVATIONS

DATE:

MY OVERALL MOOD IS:
- ○ Neutral
- ○ Curious
- ○ Irritated
- ○ Calm
- ○ Worried
- ○ Excited
- ○ Burnt Out
- ○ Preoccupied
- ○ Contemplative
- ○ Other:

THE EMOTIONS I FEEL TODAY ARE:
- ○ Happiness
- ○ Frustration
- ○ Sadness
- ○ Anger
- ○ Peace
- ○ Apathy
- ○ Overwhelm
- ○ Other:

MY BODY FEELS:
- ○ Heavy
- ○ Light
- ○ Relaxed
- ○ Alert
- ○ Grounded
- ○ Energized
- ○ Constricted
- ○ Agitated
- ○ Other:

WHAT DO I WANT TO CONTINUE NOTICING OR DOING?

WHAT INSIGHTS AND OBSERVATIONS DO I WANT TO COME BACK TO?

INSIGHTS AND OBSERVATIONS

DATE:

MY OVERALL MOOD IS:
- ○ Neutral
- ○ Curious
- ○ Irritated
- ○ Calm
- ○ Worried
- ○ Excited
- ○ Burnt Out
- ○ Preoccupied
- ○ Contemplative
- ○ Other:

THE EMOTIONS I FEEL TODAY ARE:
- ○ Happiness
- ○ Frustration
- ○ Sadness
- ○ Anger
- ○ Peace
- ○ Apathy
- ○ Overwhelm
- ○ Other:

MY BODY FEELS:
- ○ Heavy
- ○ Light
- ○ Relaxed
- ○ Alert
- ○ Grounded
- ○ Energized
- ○ Constricted
- ○ Agitated
- ○ Other:

WHAT DO I WANT TO CONTINUE NOTICING OR DOING?

WHAT INSIGHTS AND OBSERVATIONS DO I WANT TO COME BACK TO?

AFTERWORD

The wisdom and insights that can come from microdosing are lessons that you can carry with you. You may want to return to specific weeks of this journal or revisit particular prompts that resonated for you. Or maybe you're curious to take what you've learned from microdosing and apply it to other kinds of psychedelic odysseys.

Taking a macrodose or a minidose creates a perceptual change in your consciousness state. It requires a commitment to preparing a safe physical and mental space, and clear expectations and intentions. Attention to set and setting, or the circumstances of your journey, can mean the difference between a therapeutic experience and one where everything feels too uncontrolled and you can't track your insights. A macrodose or minidose of a psychedelic may deeply affect your state of being.

If you choose to explore these approaches, we suggest you prepare an environment where you will not be interrupted by the needs of the outside world during your journey. By creating a safe container, you create the conditions to go inward more easily while the psychedelic turns the knobs of your neurobiology up or down. During this time, the lid of the default mode network (see page 15) might come off completely. So clear your schedule of obligations in the hours you plan to journey and, ideally, on the following day so you can integrate your experience.

The macrodose and minidose are different tools that you can use for different purposes. A minidose creates a perceptual change, and its effects will last longer than a microdose. It will engage you in a nonordinary consciousness state for a few hours. A macrodose will be more intense and might last four to eight hours or longer. Do your research, and only increase dosage if you have the right supports set up to do so. Go slowly. Talk to trusted and knowledgeable allies. Apply the lessons about preparation, support, processing, and integration you learned from guiding your own microdosing experience.

If you journeyed with one substance for your microdose, you may be curious about the qualities of other psychedelic medicines. What are the questions and intentions that guide you to choose which substance to try next? Those who microdose with psilocybin mushrooms report a sense of ease and a loosening of tightly controlled ways of being. Those who microdose with LSD report a sharpening of perceptions and increased energy and focus. Microdosing with cannabis has been reported as resulting in a slight lift in mood. Some may microdose with ketamine or ayahuasca, among many other substances. Research the differences, and experiment responsibly.

Microdosing can set in motion a process of being in deep companionship with one's self and with others. How do you accompany yourself or others differently in your life now? In which ways are you a better companion to yourself or to others? If you went on this microdosing journey with a friend, how did this experience affect your relationship?

Small doses of awareness appeared for us in many ways. Being in conversation and companionship with one another enhanced and integrated our observations at deeper levels. We hope this journal has been *your* companion. We hope that you have felt us walking beside you on your journey.

Here are some small doses of awareness that have stayed with us:

- *Name what's elusive.*
- *Incorporate change.*
- *Explore with slow, mindful curiosity rather than fear, avoidance, or denial.*
- *Reach toward connection.*
- *Deepen friendship.*
- *Trust yourself.*
- *Be vulnerable with one another.*
- *Experiment with life.*

What small doses of awareness have stayed with you?

BIBLIOGRAPHY

Anderson, T., Petranker, R., Christopher, A., et al. (2019). Psychedelic microdosing benefits and challenges: an empirical codebook. *Harm Reduction Journal* 16(43). https://doi.org/10.1186/s12954-019-0308-4

Anderson, T., Petranker, R., Rosenbaum, D., et al. (2019). Microdosing psychedelics: personality, mental health, and creativity differences in microdosers. *Psychopharmacology* 236(2), 731–740. https://doi.org/10.1007/s00213-018-5106-2

brown, adrienne maree. (2019). *Pleasure Activism: The Politics of Feeling Good*. AK Press.

Carhart-Harris, R. L., Leech, R., Hellyer, P. J., et al. (2014). The entropic brain: a theory of conscious states informed by neuroimaging research with psychedelic drugs. *Frontiers in Human Neuroscience* 8(20). https://doi.org/10.3389/fnhum.2014.00020

Cummings, E. E. (2022). The Enormous Room. *The New York Review of Books*.

Fadiman, James. (2011). *The Psychedelic Explorer's Guide: Safe, Therapeutic, and Sacred Journeys*. Simon & Schuster.

Hart, Carl L. (2021). *Drug Use for Grown-Ups: Chasing Liberty in the Land of Fear*. Penguin Books.

Hoffman, Albert. (2017). *LSD, My Problem Child: Reflections on Sacred Drugs, Mysticism, and Science*, 4th edition. Multidisciplinary Association for Psychedelic Studies.

Janikian, Michelle. (2018). *Your Psilocybin Mushroom Companion: An Informative, Easy-to-Use Guide to Understanding Magic Mushrooms—From Tips and Trips to Microdosing and Psychedelic Therapy*. Ulysses Press.

Kuypers, K.P.C. (2020). The therapeutic potential of microdosing psychedelics in depression. *Therapeutic Advances in Psychopharmacology* 10: 1–15. https://doi.org/10.1177/2045125320950567

Polito, V., & Stevenson, R. J. (2019). A systematic study of microdosing psychedelics. *PloS ONE* 14(2): e0211023. https://doi.org/10.1371/journal.pone.0211023

Pollan, Michael. (February 2, 2015). The Trip Treatment. *The New Yorker*. www.newyorker.com/magazine/2015/02/09/trip-treatment

Pollan, Michael. (2019). *How to Change Your Mind*. Penguin Press.

Pollan, Michael. (2021). *This Is Your Mind on Plants*. Penguin Press.

Rootman, J. M., Kryskow, P., Harvey, K., et al. (2021). Adults who microdose psychedelics report health related motivations and lower levels of anxiety and depression compared to non-microdosers. *Scientific Reports* 11(22479). https://doi.org/10.1038/s41598-021-01811-4

Stamets, Paul. (2005). *Mycelium Running: How Mushrooms Can Help Save the World*. Ten Speed Press.

Waldman, Ayelet. (2017). *A Really Good Day: How Microdosing Made a Mega Difference in My Mood, My Marriage, and My Life*. Knopf Doubleday.

Williams, Wendy. (2020). *The Language of Butterflies: How Thieves, Hoarders, Scientists, and Other Obsessives Unlocked the Secrets of the World's Favorite Insect*. Simon & Schuster.

Winnicott, D.W. (1960). Ego distortion in terms of true and false self. In Winnicott, D.W., ed., *The Maturational Processes and the Facilitating Environment: Studies in the Theory of Emotional Development*. Karnac Books, 140–152.

Yeshurun, Y., Nguyen, M., & Hasson, U. (2021). The default mode network: where the idiosyncratic self meets the shared social world. *Nature Reviews Neuroscience*, 22(3), 181–192. https://doi.org/10.1038/s41583-020-00420-w

RESOURCES

The following short list of curated resources, although not comprehensive, primarily highlights women- and BIPOC-led affinity groups and resources that spotlight underrepresented communities. Many resources for psychedelic-assisted therapy or facilitator training exist, including programs at Naropa University and California Institute of Integral Studies. Amy Wong Hope is a psychotherapist by profession. She's not your psychotherapist. Use of this book does not create any kind of therapist-client relationship. Always consult with a professional for your specific needs and circumstances prior to making any medical or legal decisions. This list includes national and international mainstream informational resources along with resources and informational hubs that may be lesser known.

ALMA INSTITUTE
www.almatraining.org

ASIAN PSYCHEDELIC COLLECTIVE
www.asianpsychedeliccollective.org

BECKLEY FOUNDATION: MICRODOSING
www.beckleyfoundation.org/microdosing

CHACRUNA INSTITUTE FOR PSYCHEDELIC PLANT MEDICINES
https://chacruna.net

FUNGI FOUNDATION
www.ffungi.org

JOHNS HOPKINS PSYCHEDELICS RESEARCH AND PSILOCYBIN THERAPY
www.hopkinsmedicine.org/psychiatry/research/psychedelics-research.html

***THE MICRODOSE* (A NEWSLETTER FROM THE UC BERKELEY CENTER FOR THE SCIENCE OF PSYCHEDELICS)**
https://themicrodose.substack.com

MICRODOSE.ME (AFFILIATED WITH THE UNIVERSITY OF BRITISH COLUMBIA AND PAUL STAMETS)
https://microdose.me

MICRODOSING INSTITUTE
https://microdosinginstitute.com

MULTIDISCIPLINARY ASSOCIATION FOR PSYCHEDELIC STUDIES
http://maps.org

PEOPLE OF COLOR PSYCHEDELIC COLLECTIVE
www.pocpc.org

PLANT PARENTHOOD
www.plantph.com

PSYCHEDELIC ALPHA: PSYCHEDELIC LEGALIZATION & DECRIMINALIZATION TRACKER
https://psychedelicalpha.com/data/psychedelic-laws

PSYCHEDELIC LIBERATION COLLECTIVE
https://psychedelicliberationcollective.com

ABOUT THE AUTHORS

Shin Yu Pai is an award-winning author, visual artist, and teacher of creative writing. Shin Yu has published eleven books, including most recently the poetry collection *Virga* (Empty Bowl, 2021). She is currently Civic Poet of Seattle (2023–2024). In 2020, Entre Rios Books published *Ensō*, a survey spanning twenty years of Shin Yu's work across creative disciplines including photography, book arts, poetry, and personal essays. She received her MFA from the School of the Art Institute of Chicago and has taught at Northwest Film Forum, Henry Art Gallery, Dallas Museum of Art, and other creative institutions. She is a 2022 Artist Trust Fellow and was short-listed in 2014 for a Stranger Genius Award in Literature. Shin Yu has been a practicing Buddhist for twenty-five years and studied contemplative practice and mindfulness at Naropa University, where she earned a certificate in Authentic Leadership. Currently, she is the host, writer, and producer of *The Ten Thousand Things*, a podcast on Asian American stories for KUOW Public Radio, Seattle's NPR affiliate station.

Amy Wong Hope is a licensed clinical social worker and Program Certificate Director for the Psychedelics Studies program at the New Earth Institute at Southwestern College in Santa Fe, New Mexico. She has a private psychotherapy practice focusing on evidence-based practices that support resolving the effects of trauma on neurobiology and attachment styles and restoring resiliency in her clients' lives. She completed her postgraduate fellowship at the Trauma Center at JRI in Boston, and she is an Albert Schweitzer Fellow for Life. She has advanced training in EMDR, Sensorimotor Psychotherapy, Brainspotting, Internal Family Systems, and mindfulness. Amy is an MDMA-Assisted Therapy therapist trained through the Multidisciplinary Association for Psychedelic Studies (MAPS), and she holds a Diversity, Culture and Social Justice in Psychedelics certification from Chacruna Institute and an MSW from Simmons College.

ACKNOWLEDGMENTS

Thank you to Yingzhao Liu for hosting us at her Original Mind Residency, where the majority of the book was written and edited.

We wish to express our thanks to Jennifer Worick and Sharyn Rosart for their enthusiasm and early support of this project when it was just an inkling of an idea. Gratitude is also due to Karen Maeda Allman and Elizabeth Wales for their advice and literary counsel. You really helped us understand the landscape and context for this project. Thanks to Allison Adler and the Chronicle team.

The authors are grateful to Melanie Noel, Stephen Robinson, Preeti Sethi, Gerry Valentine, and Heike Karsch for reading early drafts of this project.

SHIN YU

I am grateful to my therapist, Bob, for being there to undo the loneliness. My work would not have been possible without the support of my partner, Kort. Lastly, I express thanks for friend and co-author Amy Wong Hope, who brought pleasure and care to the writing of this book.

AMY

I am thankful to facilitators, past and present, for holding space through the years for my real self to step forward rather than my conditioned parts. I am grateful for the support and encouragement of my husband, Ethan, who supports me in my authenticity and reminds me to take breaks. Thank you to the many dear friends who have helped me dance with my shadow and trust my strengths; to my mother, Nancy, for her nonjudgmental and loving support; and to my brother, Dean, who I laugh with about life's cosmic jokes. Lastly, I wish to thank Shin Yu for asking me to collaborate on this project. I wasn't sure I was ready to work so closely with anybody, but I found the experience illuminating, connecting, exciting, fun, and pleasurable; and it reaffirmed my belief that true collaboration is possible.

Copyright © 2024 by Amy Wong Hope & Shin Yu Pai.
All rights reserved. No part of this book may be reproduced in any form
without written permission from the publisher.

ISBN 978-1-7972-2782-5

Manufactured in China.

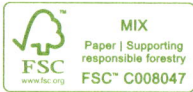

Design by Natalie Snodgrass.
Typeset in Voir, Maison Neue, and Plantin.

This book contains advice and information relating to health and interpersonal well-being. It is not intended to replace medical or psychotherapeutic advice and should be used to supplement rather than replace any needed care by your doctor or mental health professional. While all efforts have been made to ensure the accuracy of the information contained in this book as of the date of publication, the publisher and the author are not responsible for any adverse effects or consequences that may occur as a result of applying the methods suggested in this book.

10 9 8 7 6 5 4 3 2 1

Chronicle books and gifts are available at special quantity discounts to corporations, professional associations, literacy programs, and other organizations. For details and discount information, please contact our premiums department at corporatesales@chroniclebooks.com or at 1-800-759-0190.

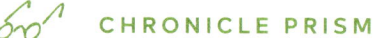 CHRONICLE PRISM

Chronicle Prism is an imprint of Chronicle Books LLC,
680 Second Street, San Francisco, California 94107

chronicleprism.com

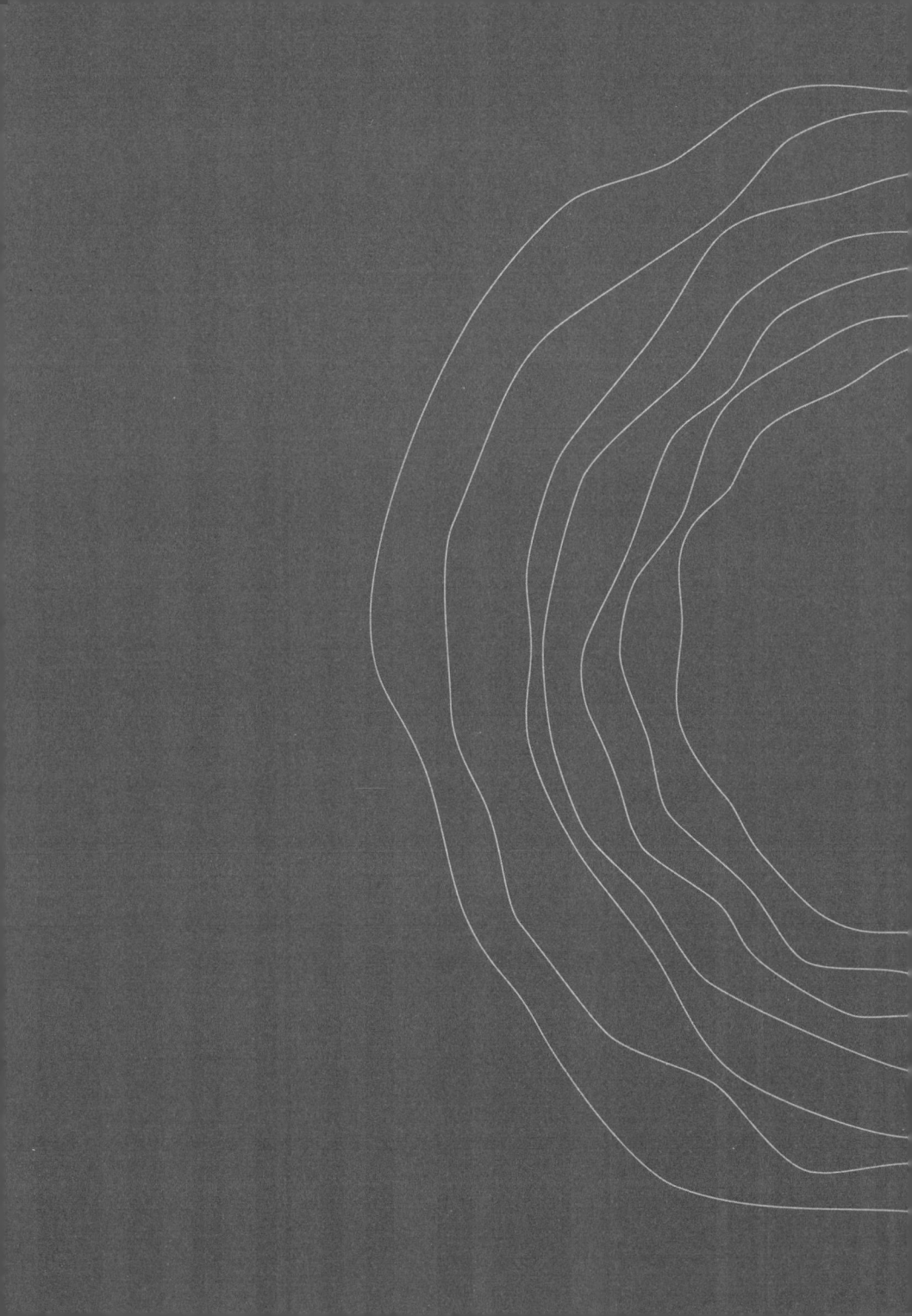